Breasts:
The Ultimate Photo Collection

By
Scarlett Belanger

www.amorouspress.com

ISBN-10: 0615485960
ISBN-13: 978-0615485966

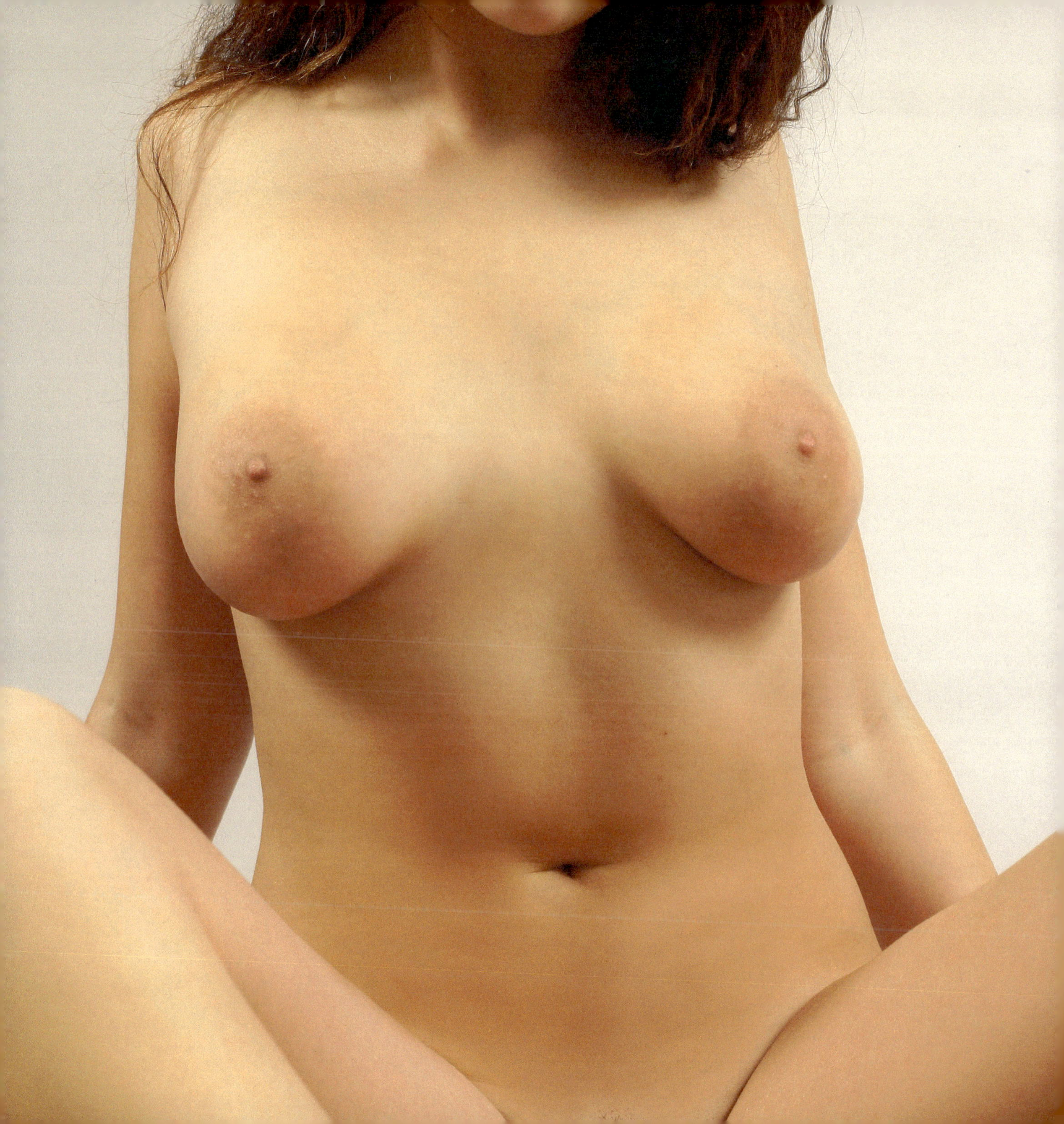

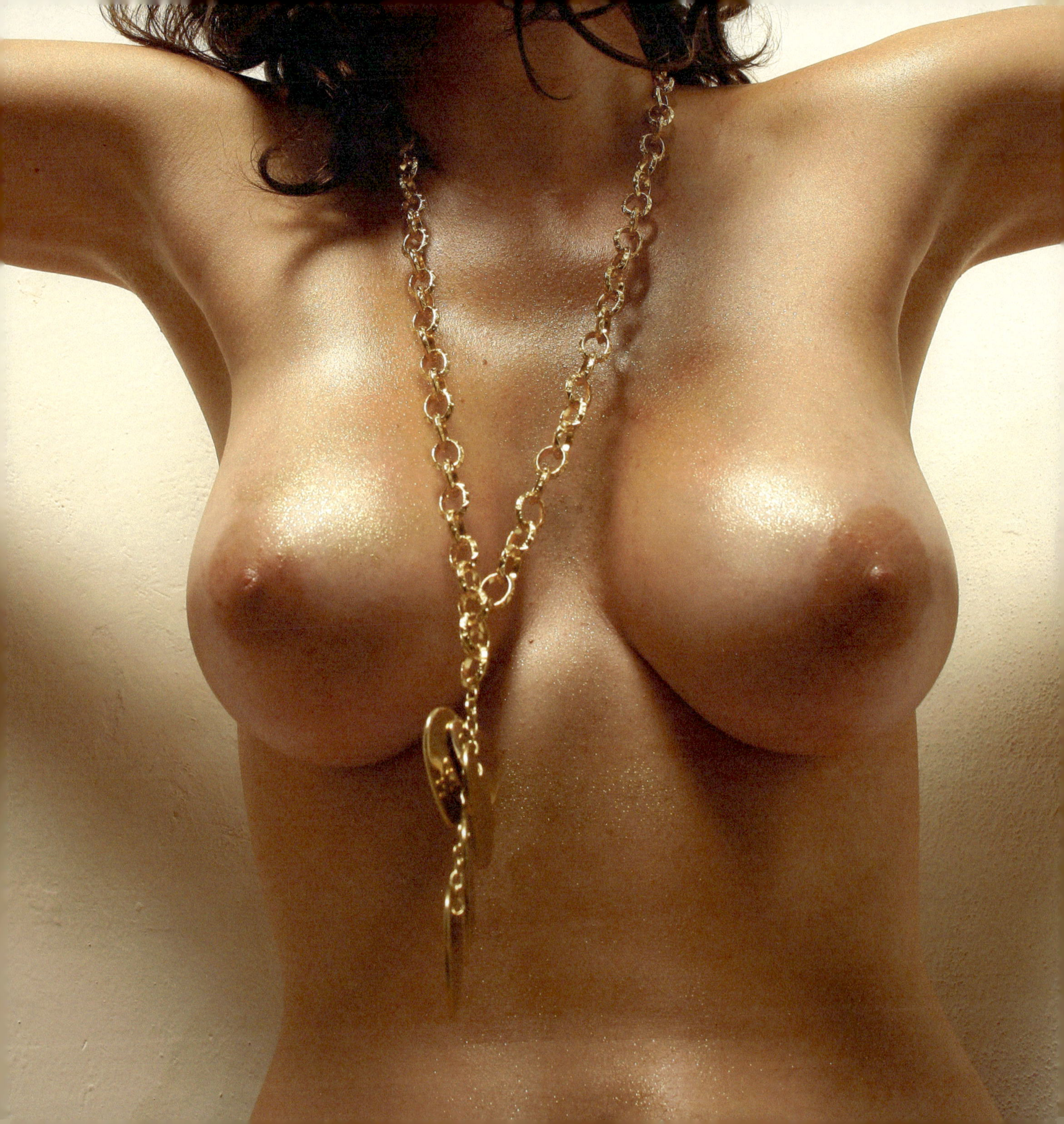

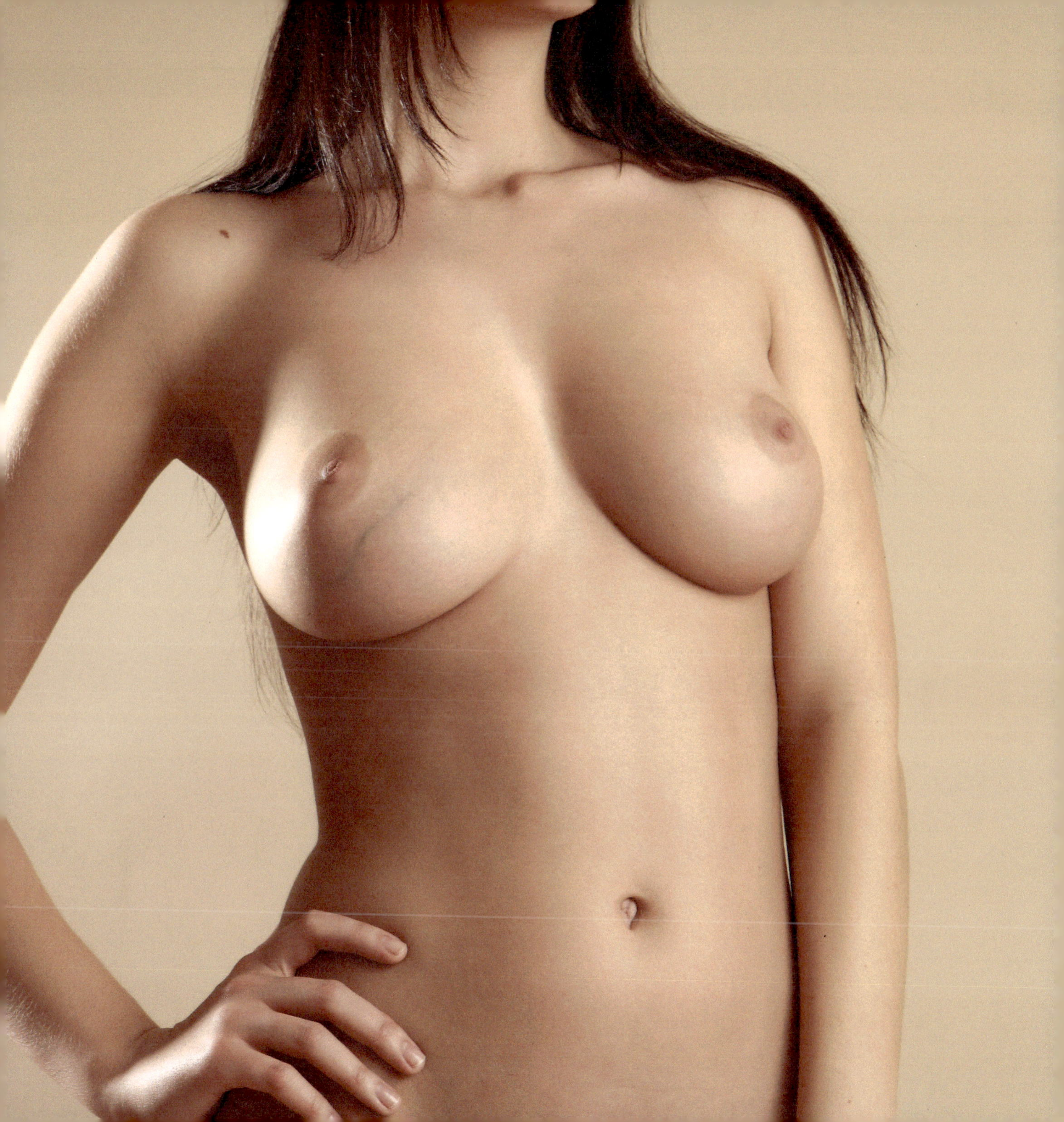

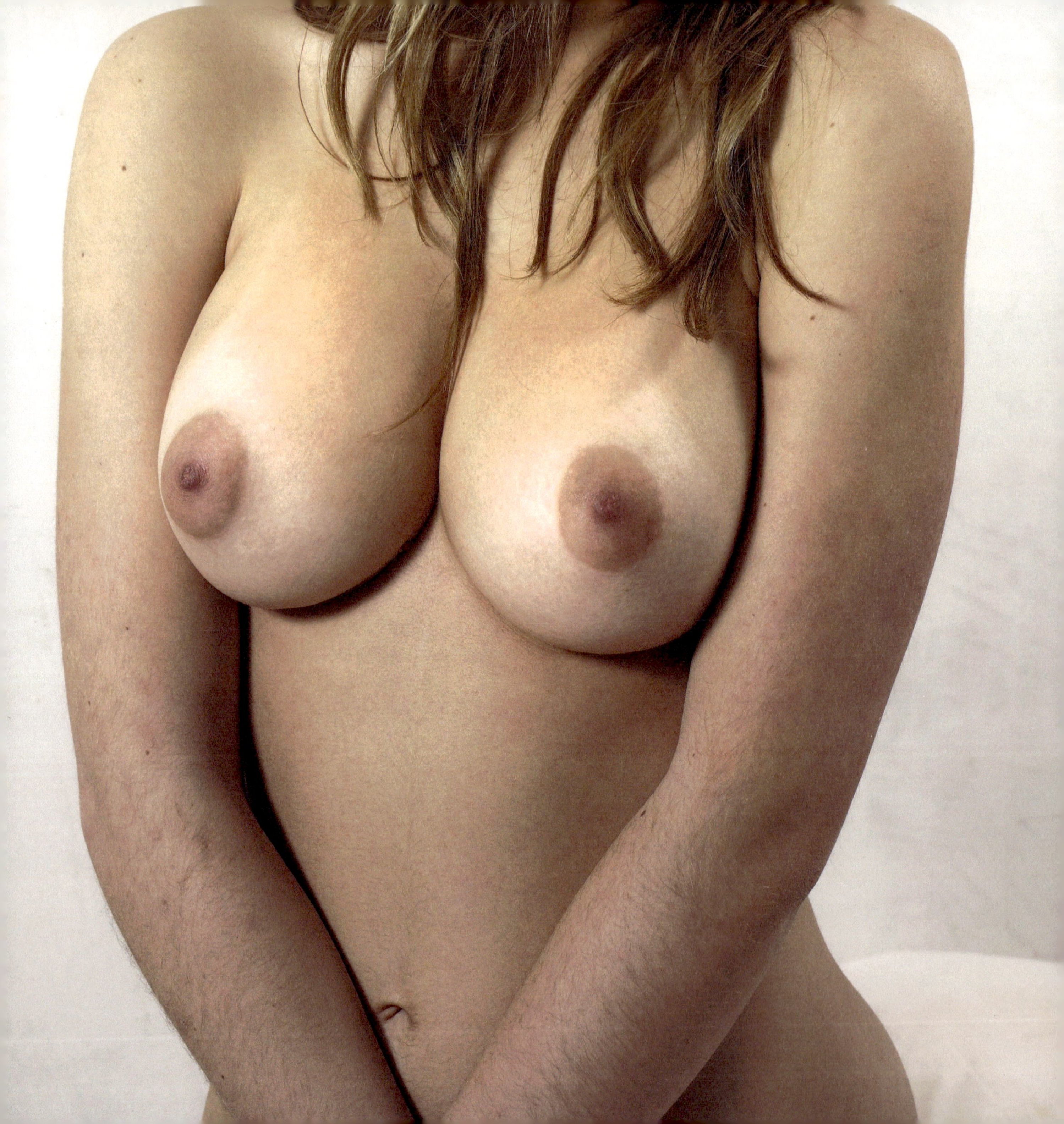

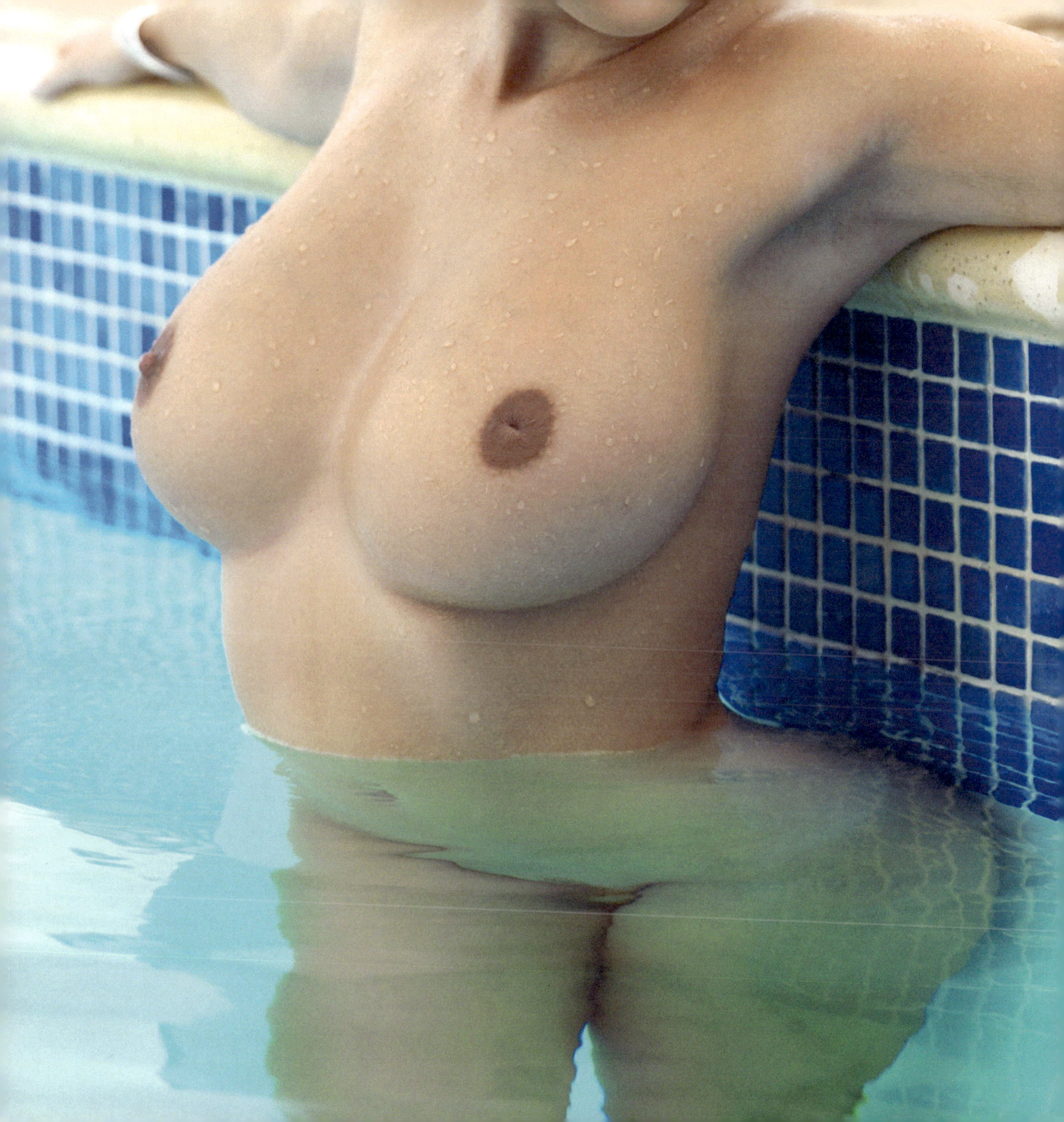

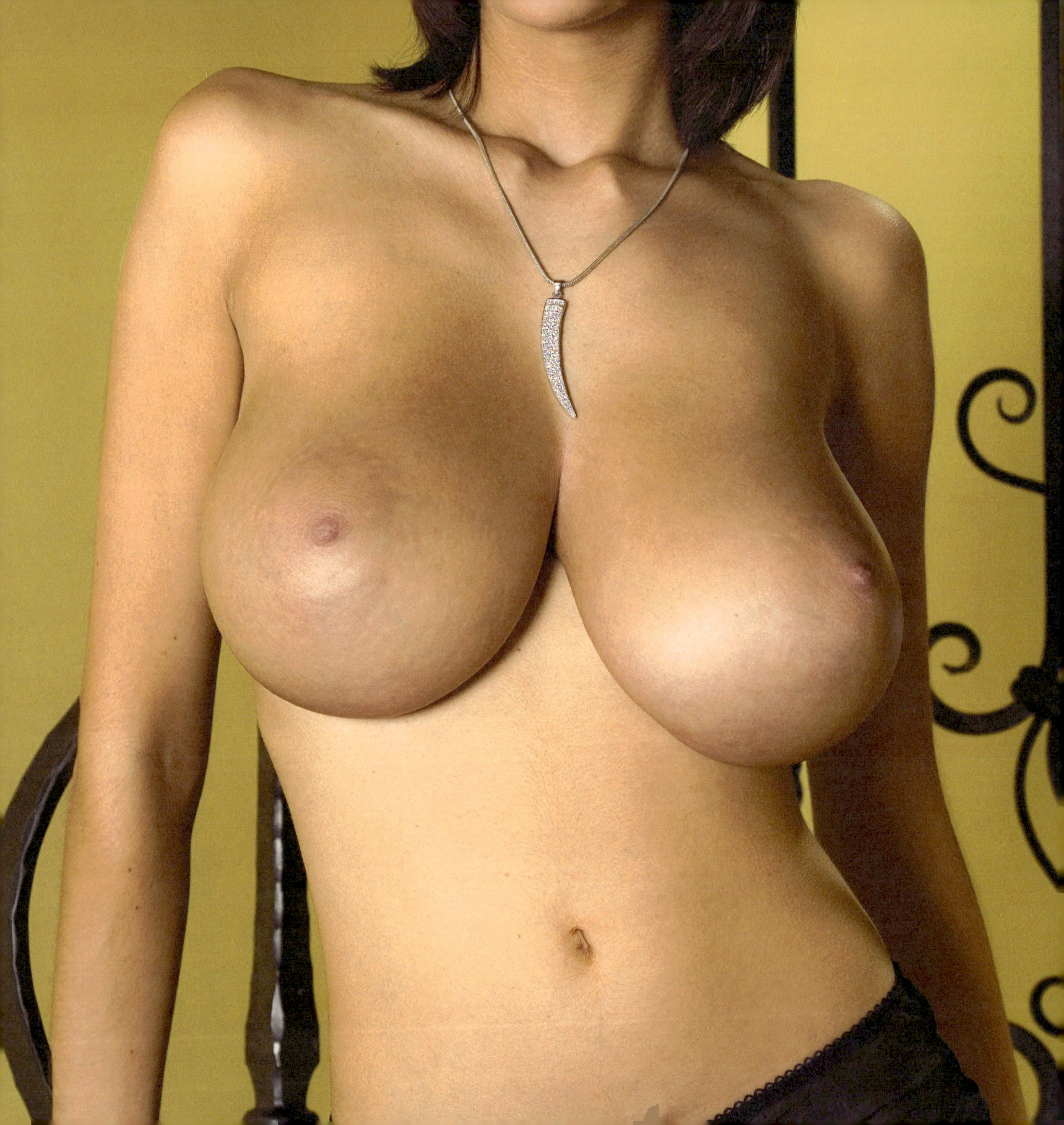

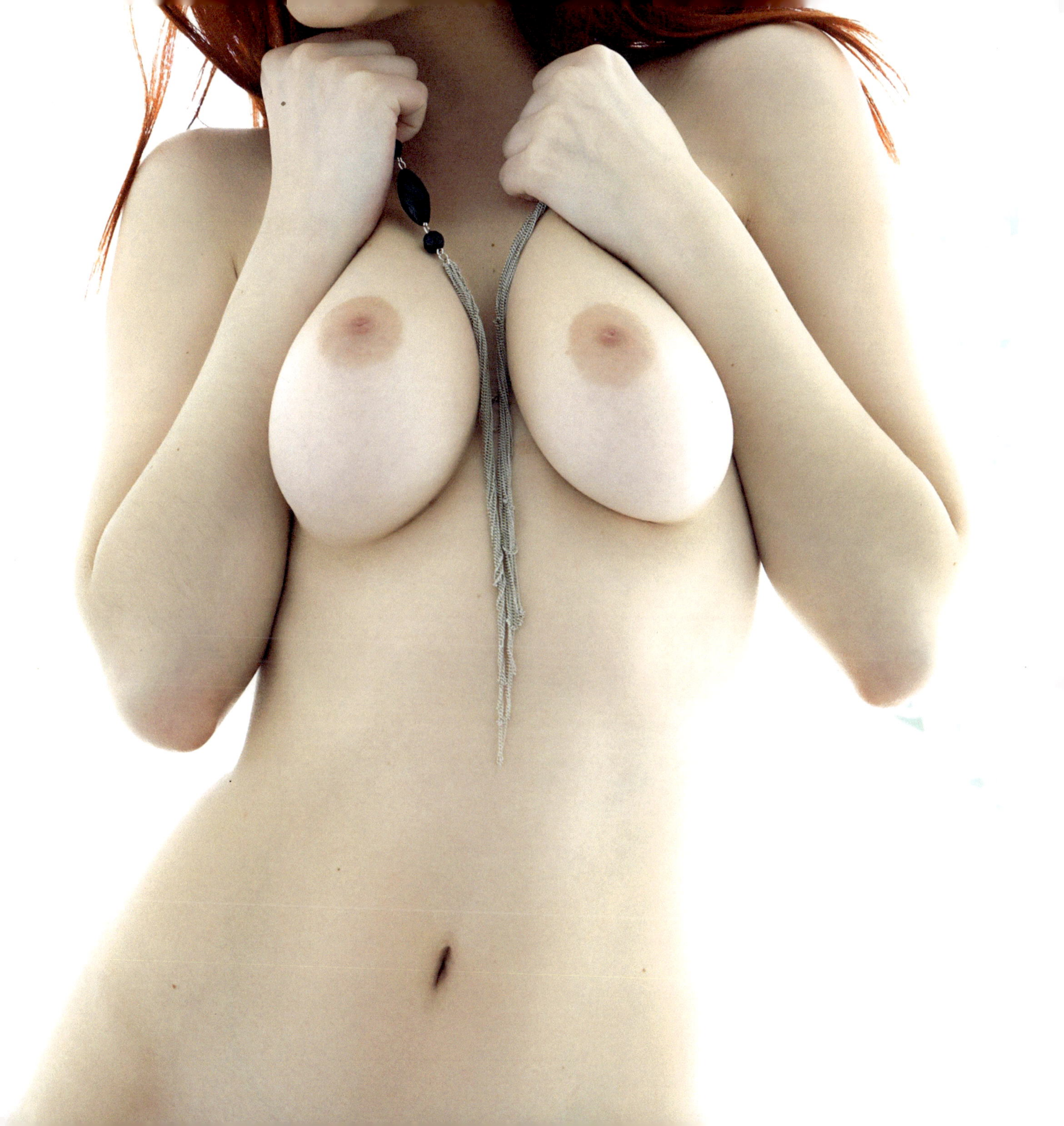

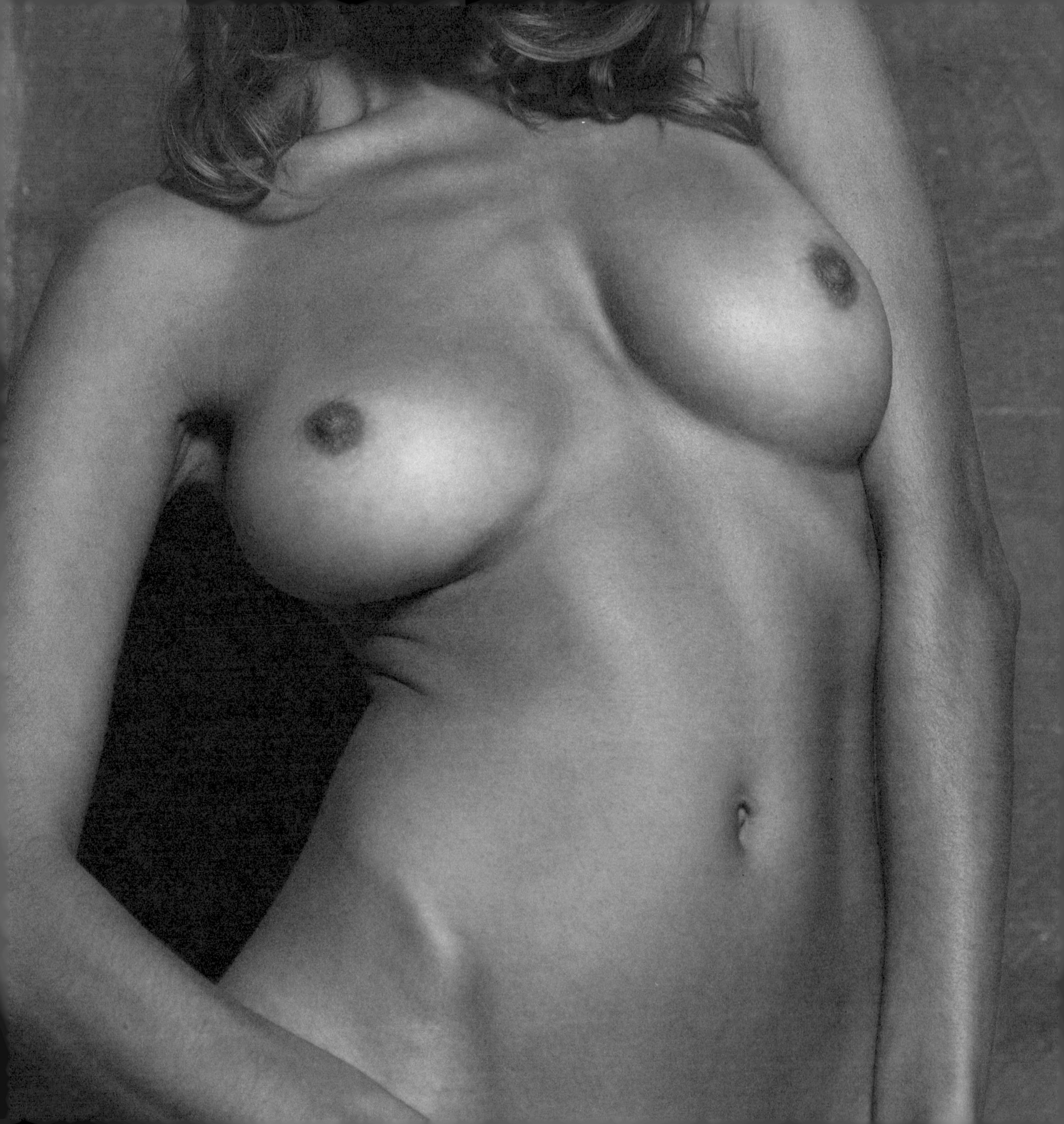

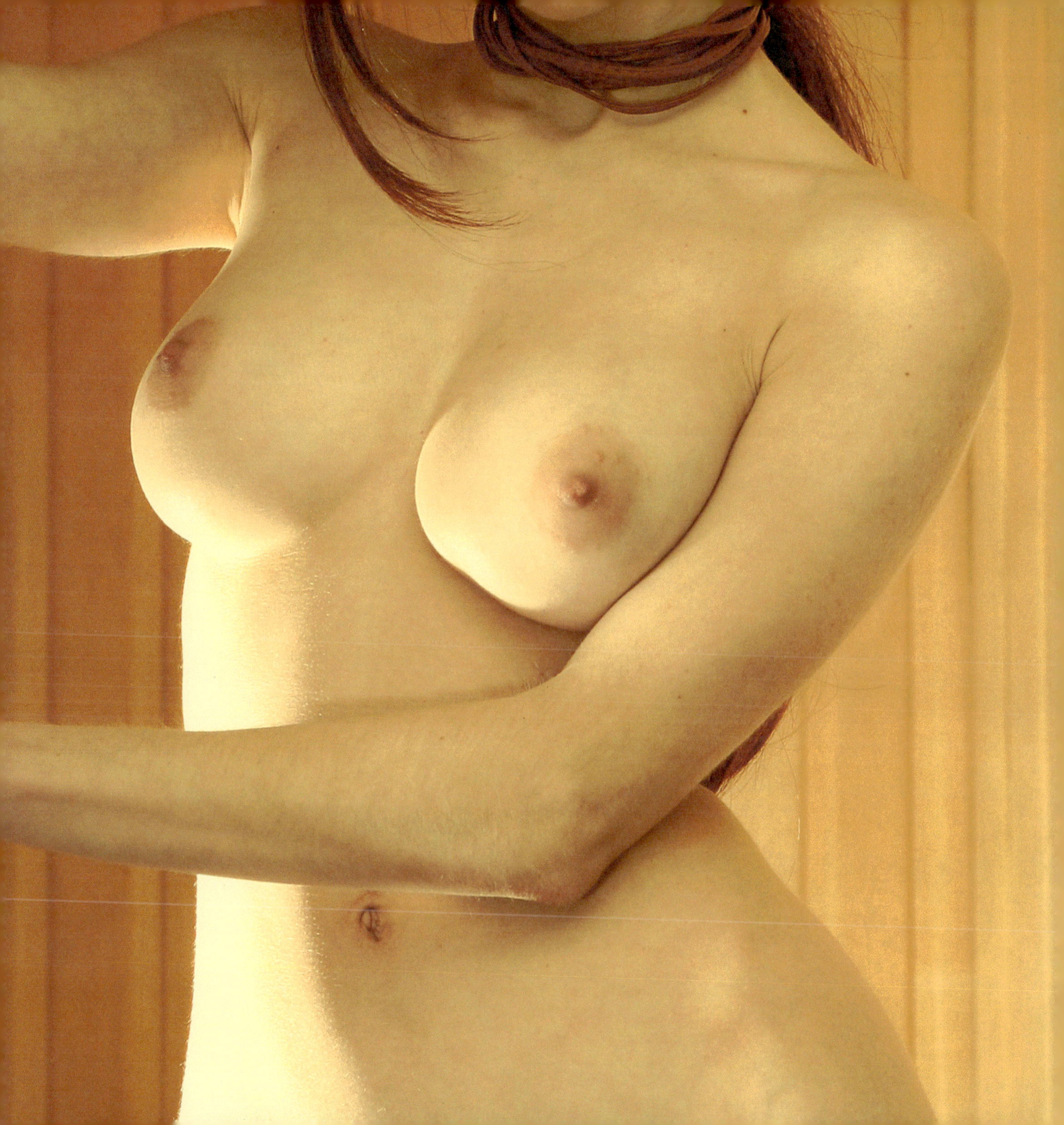

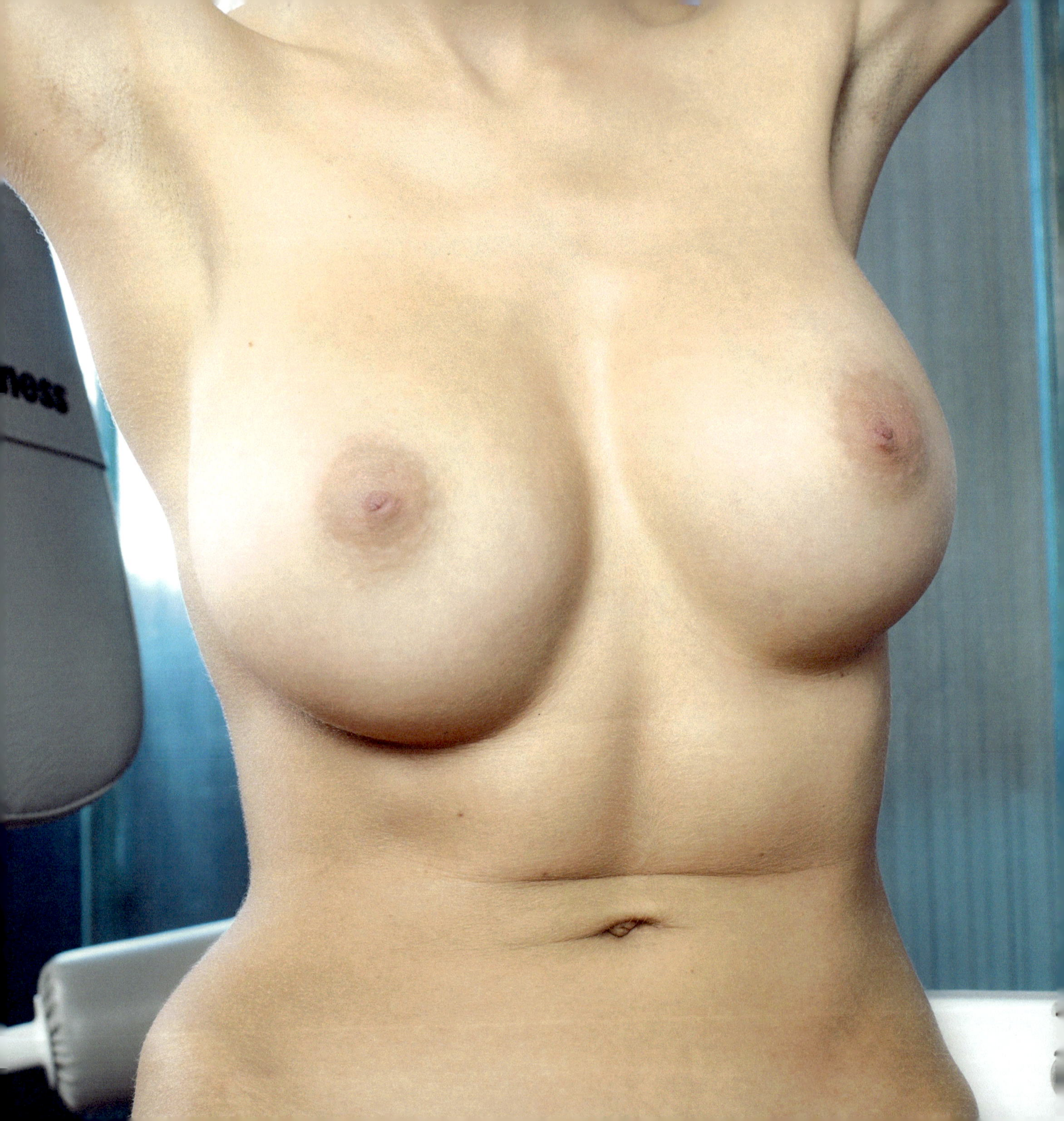

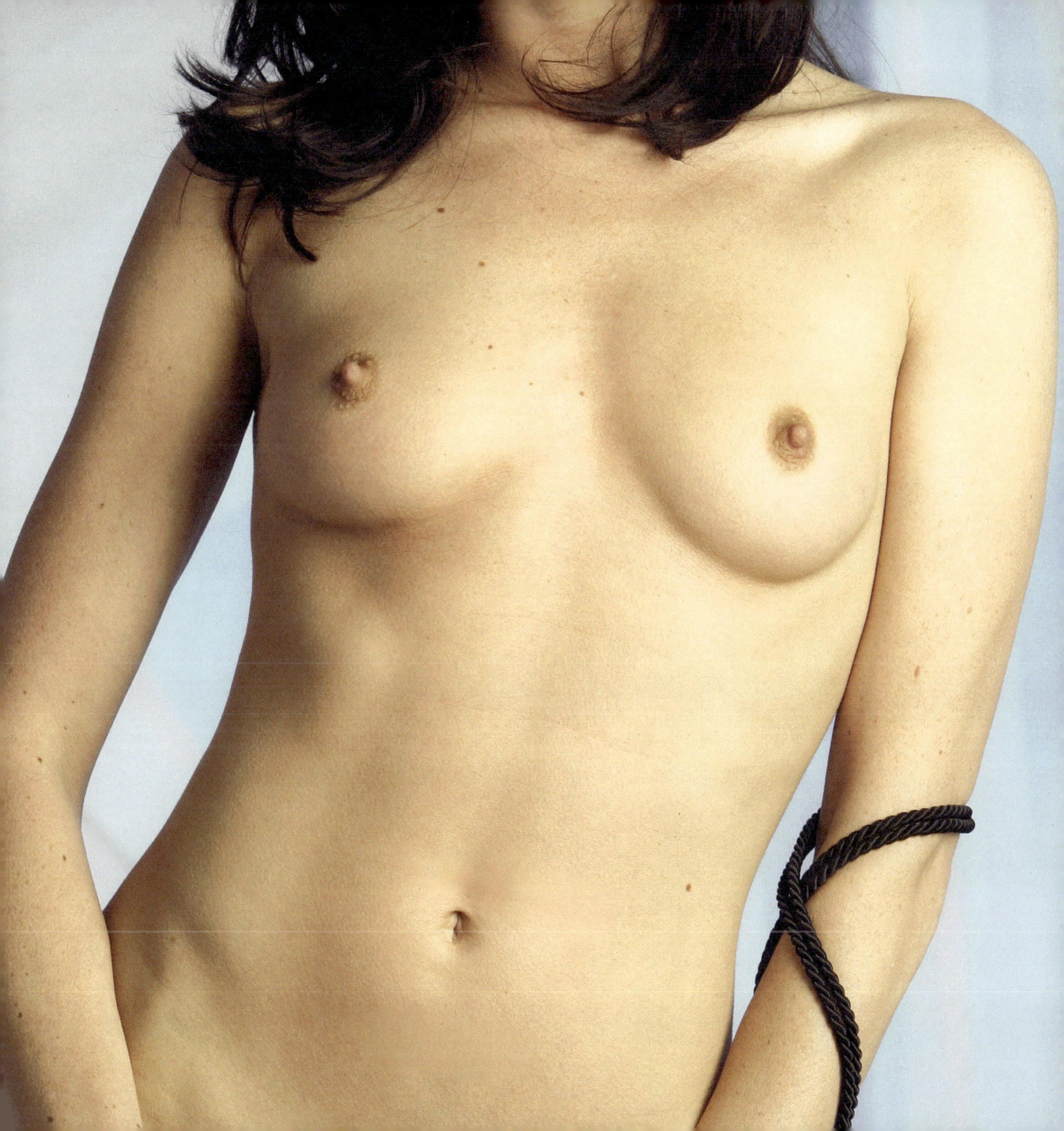

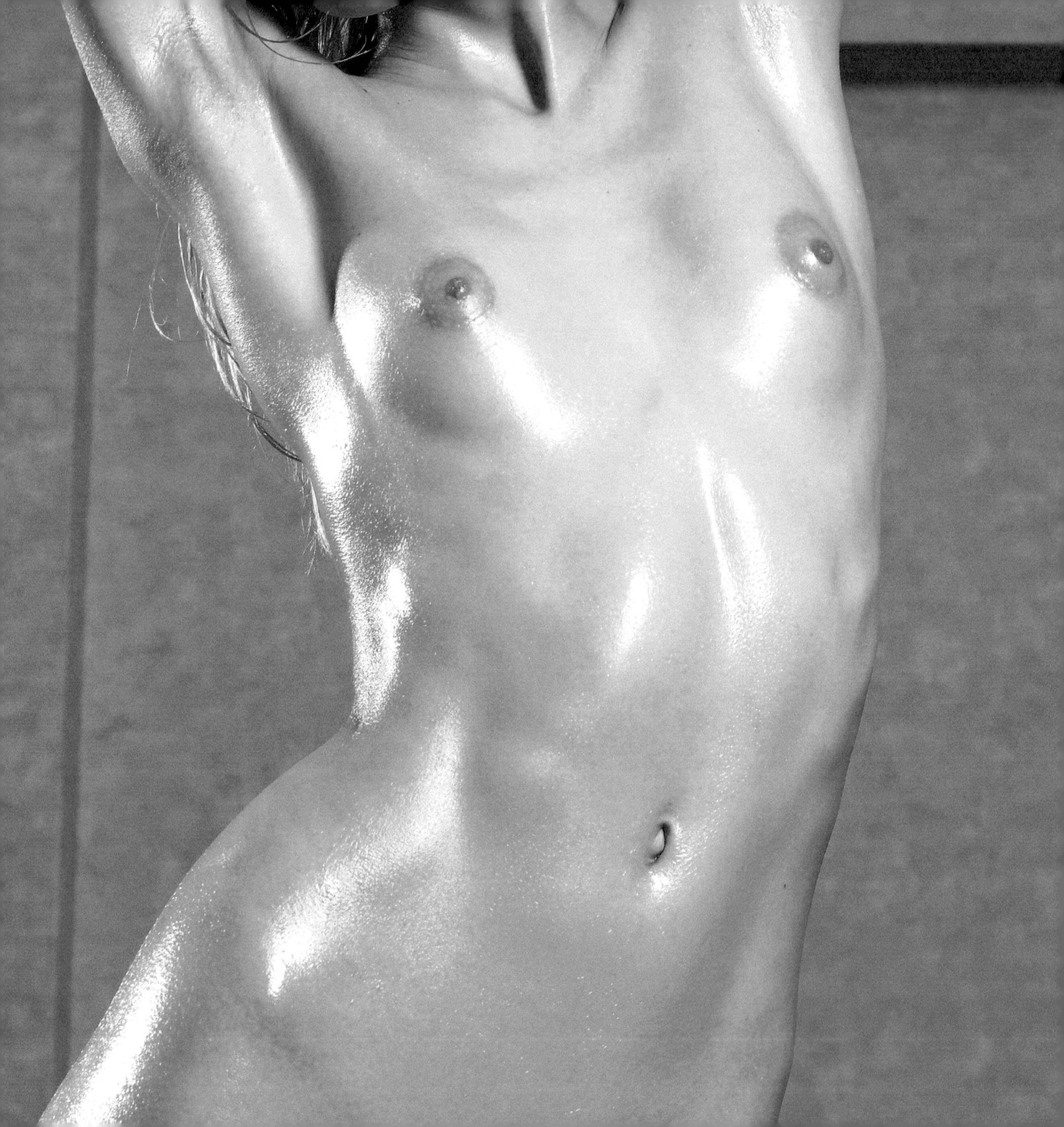

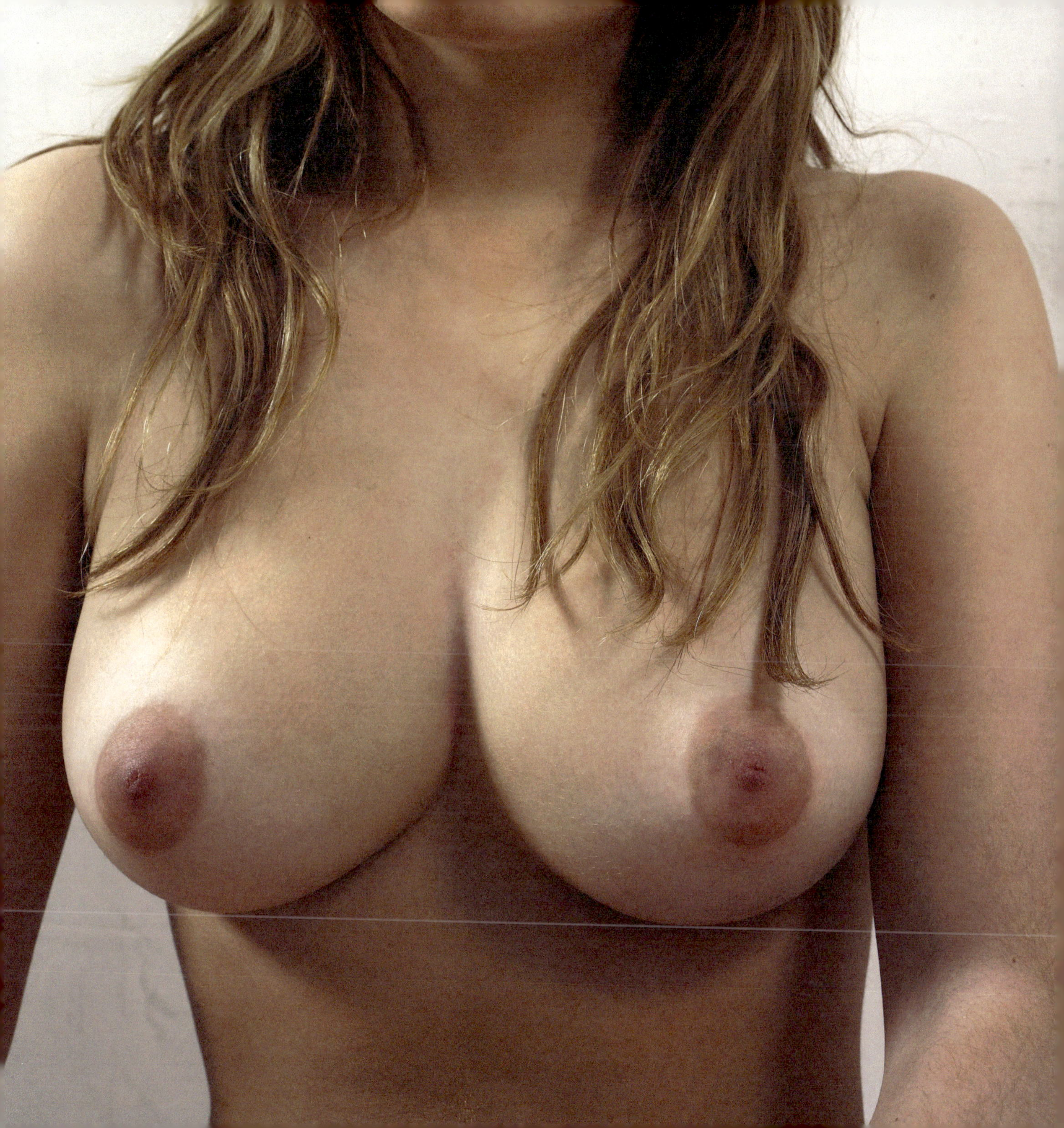

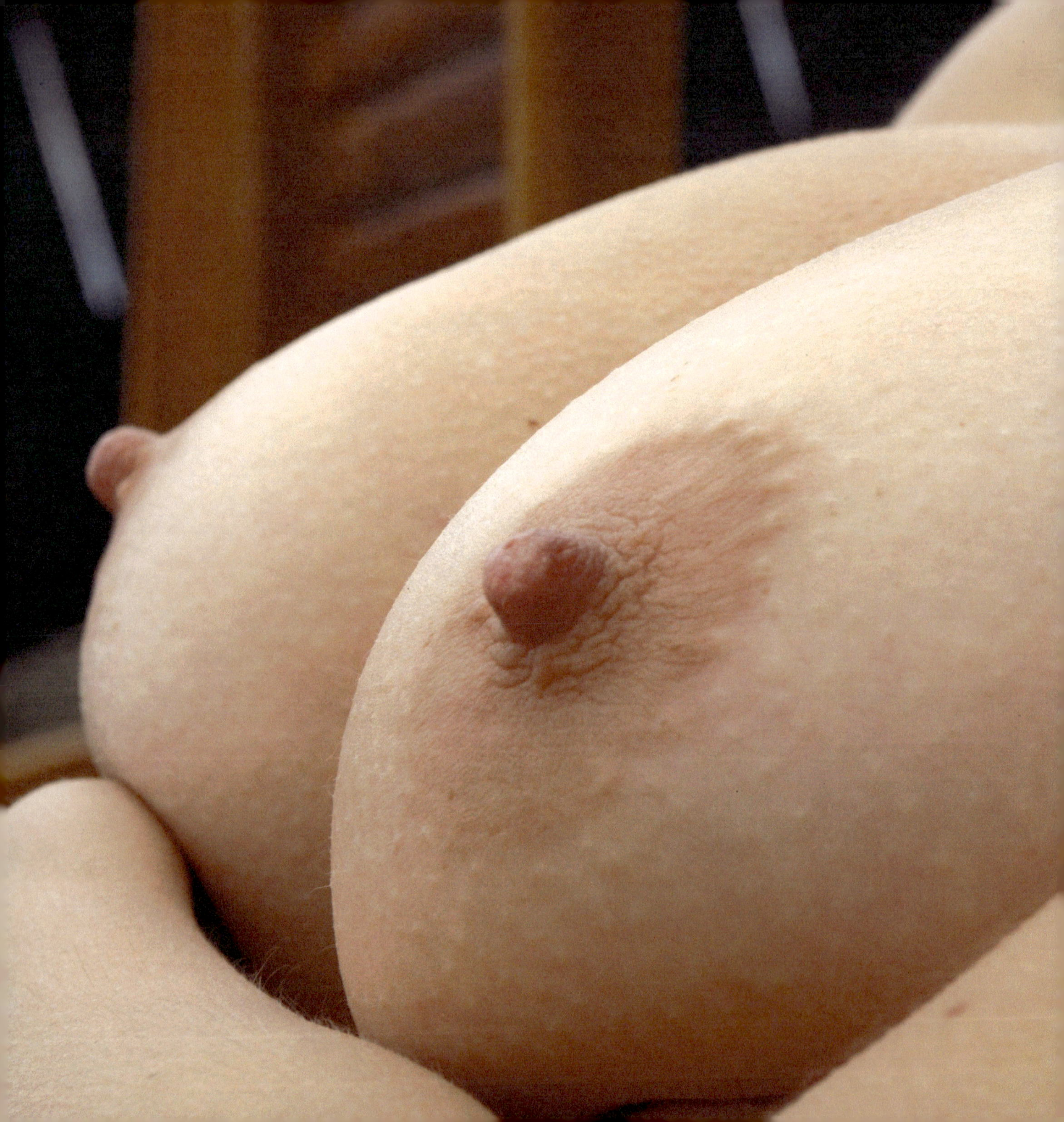

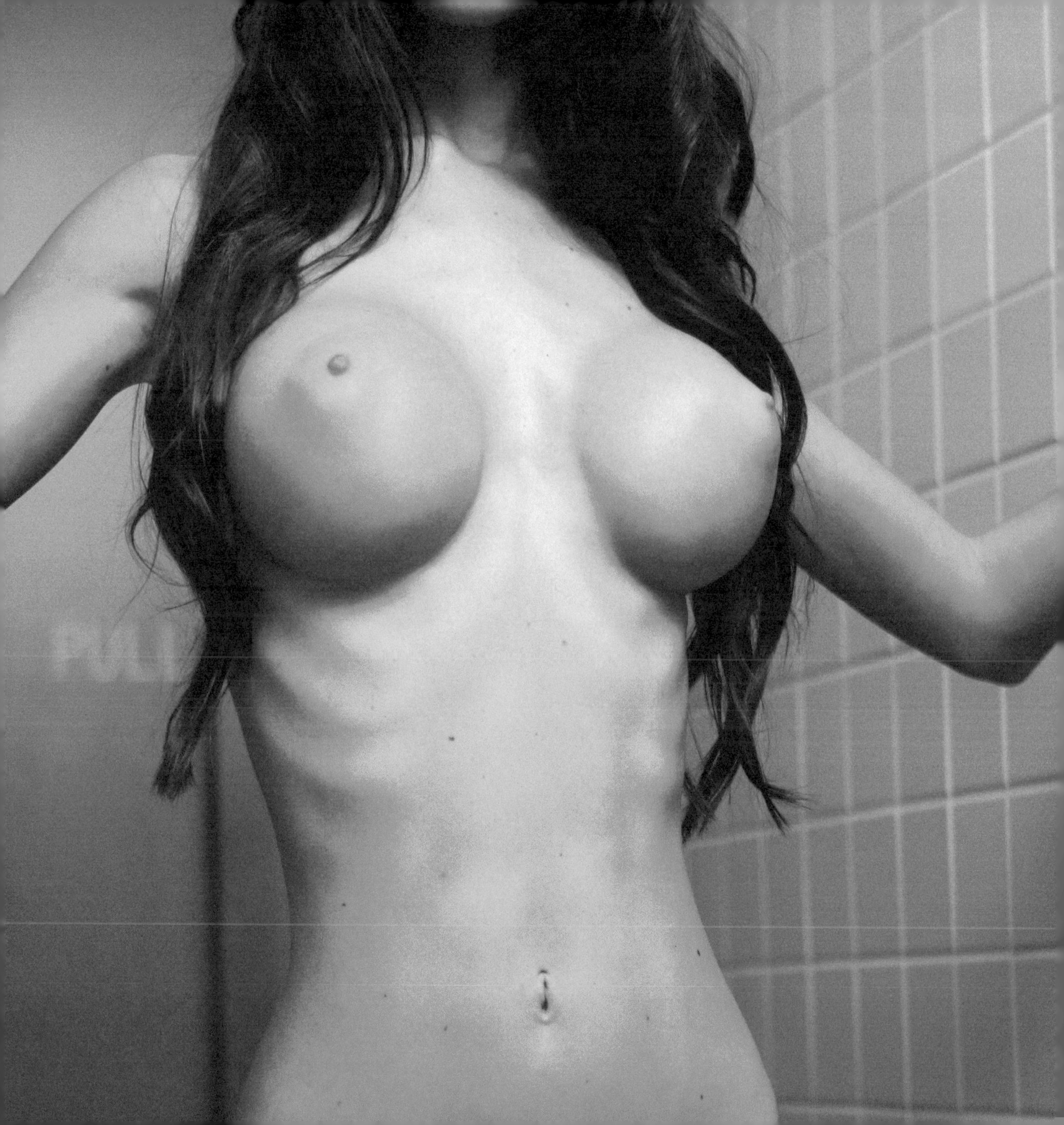

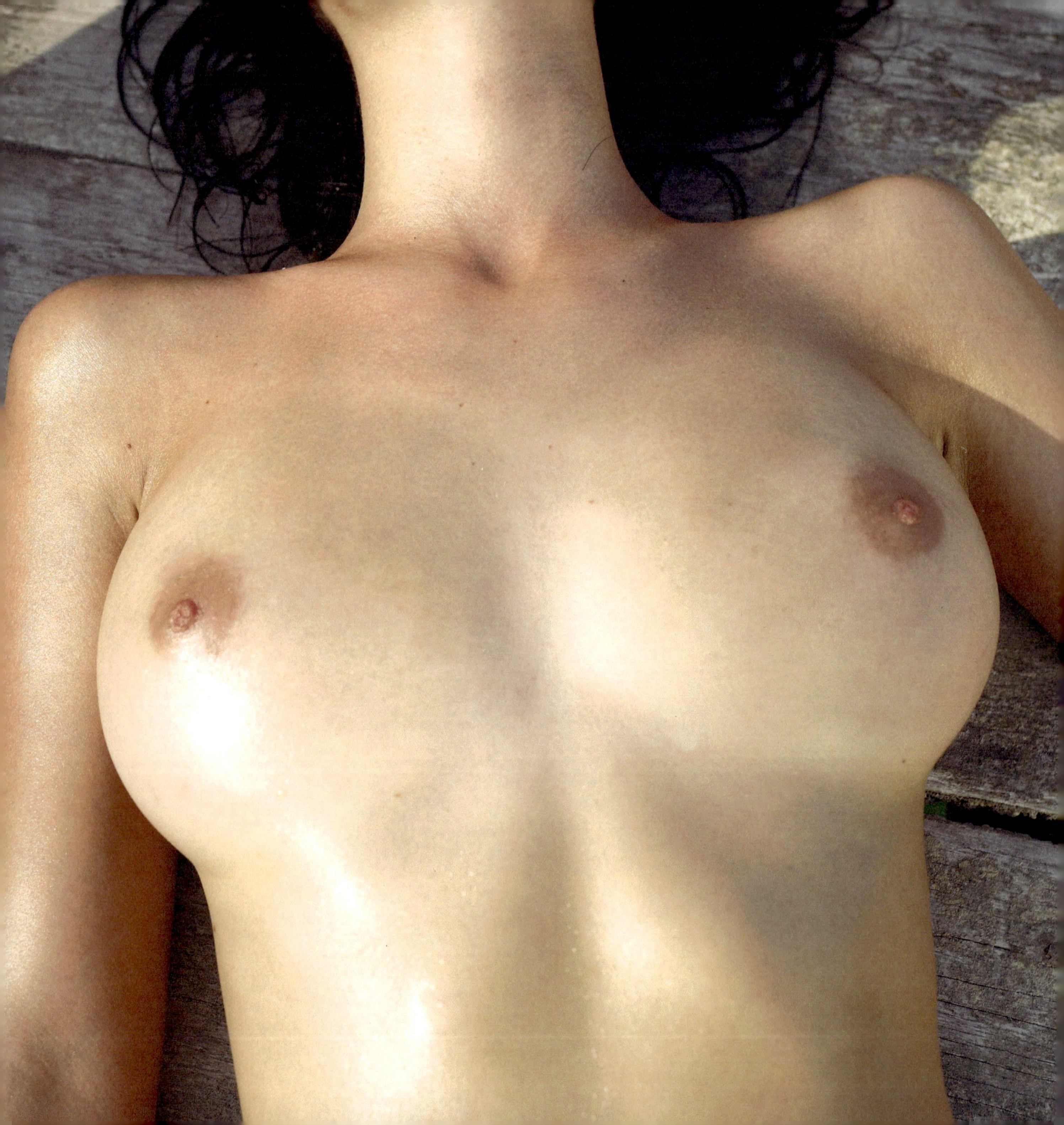

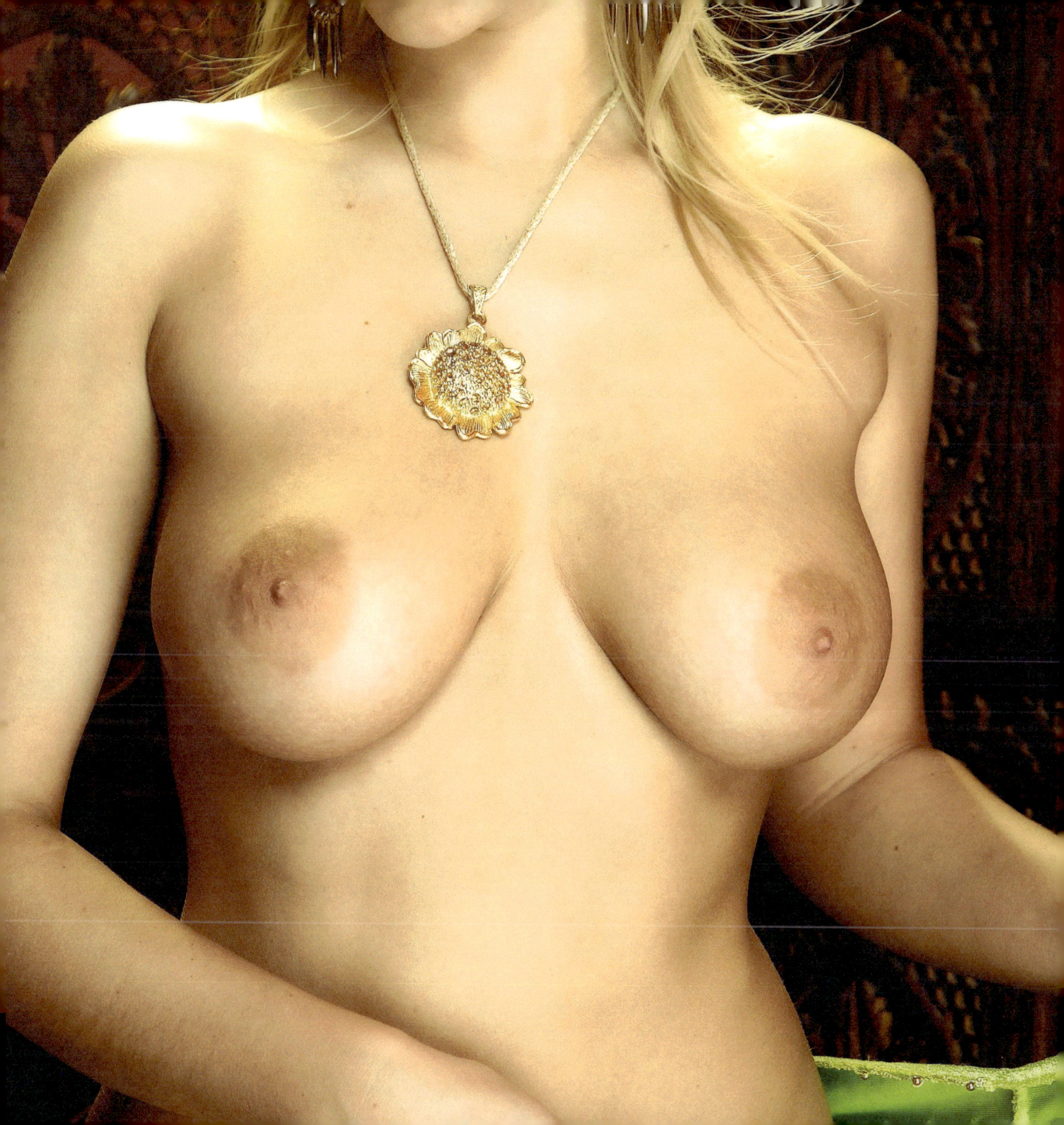

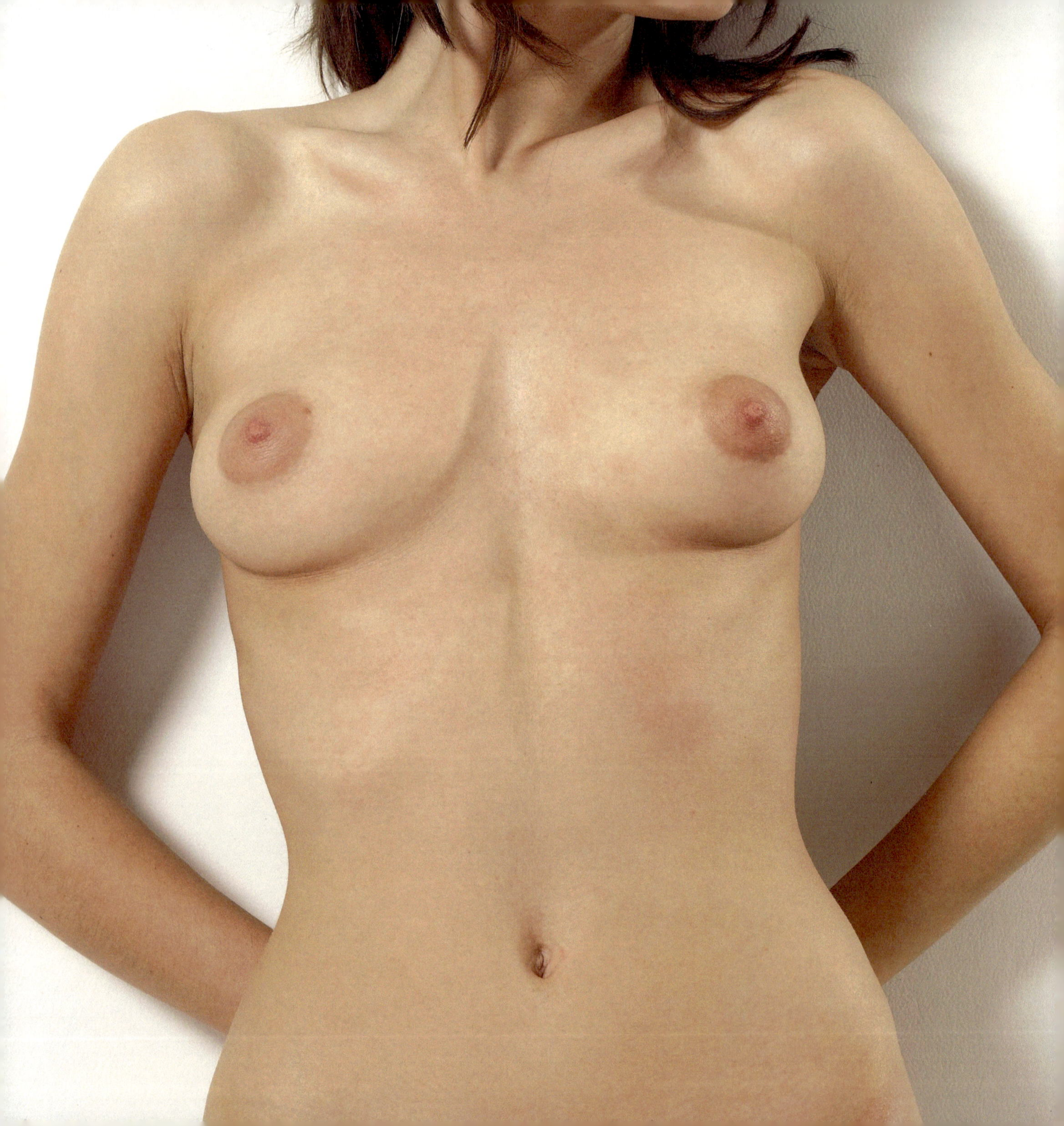

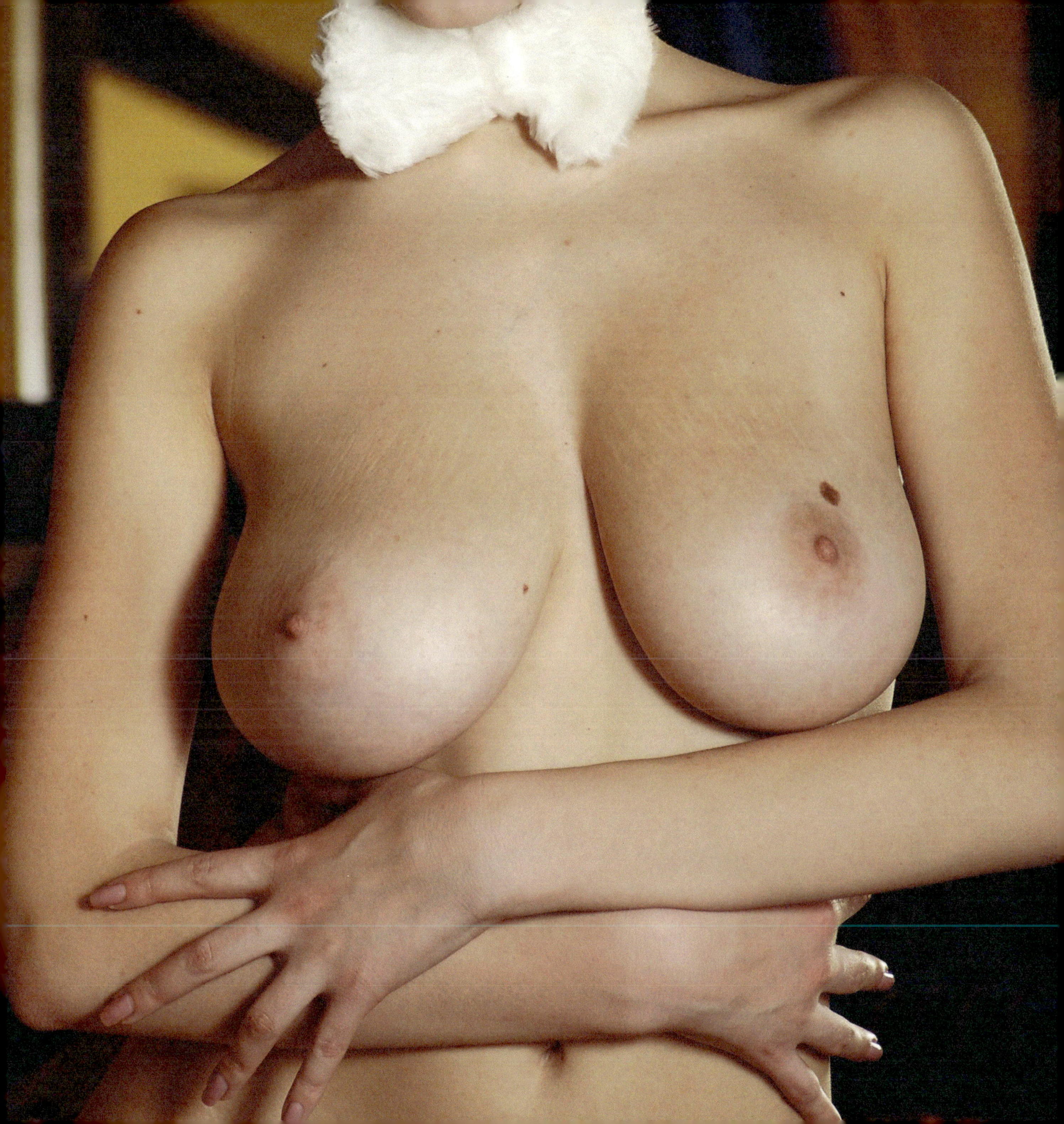

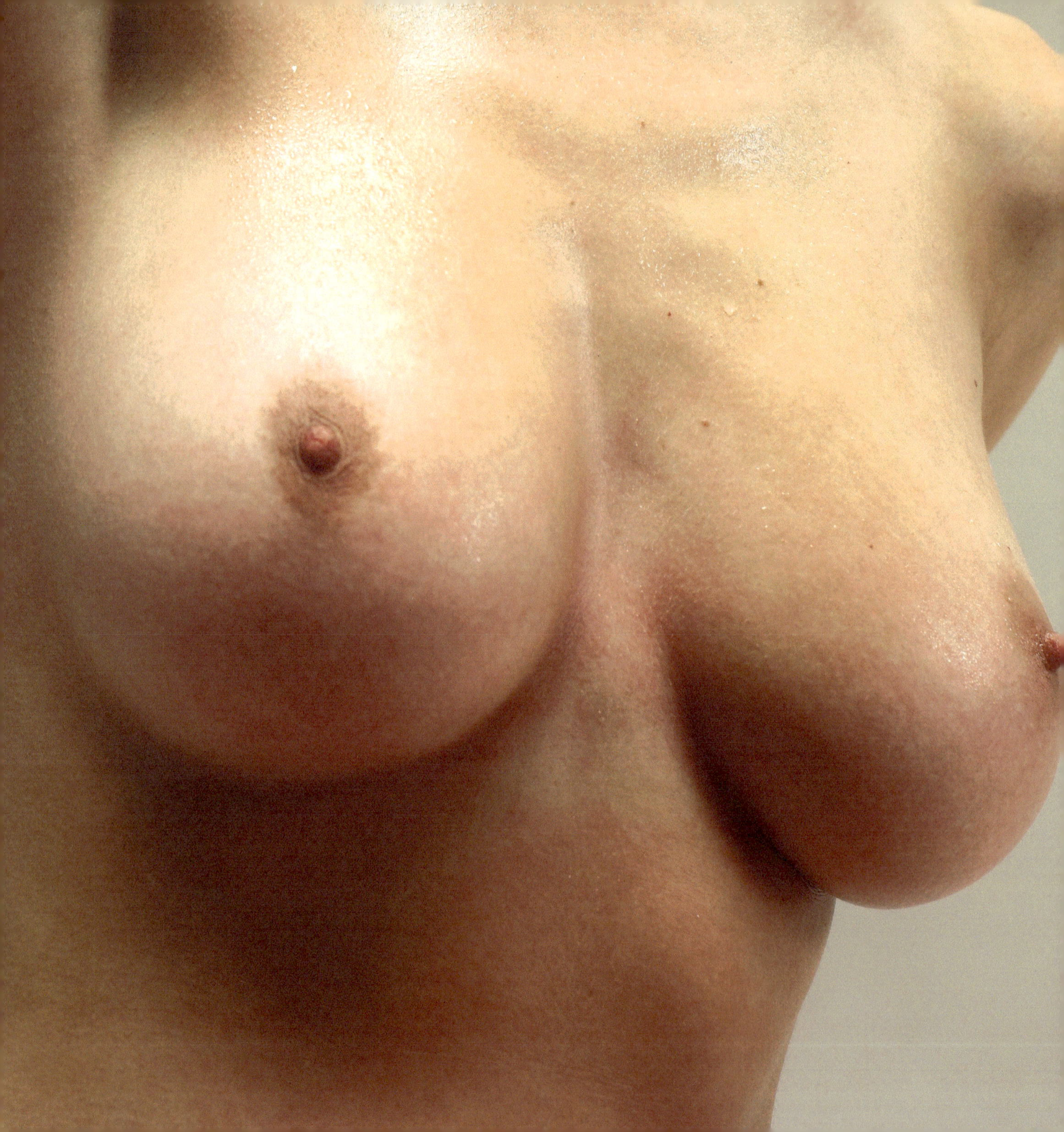

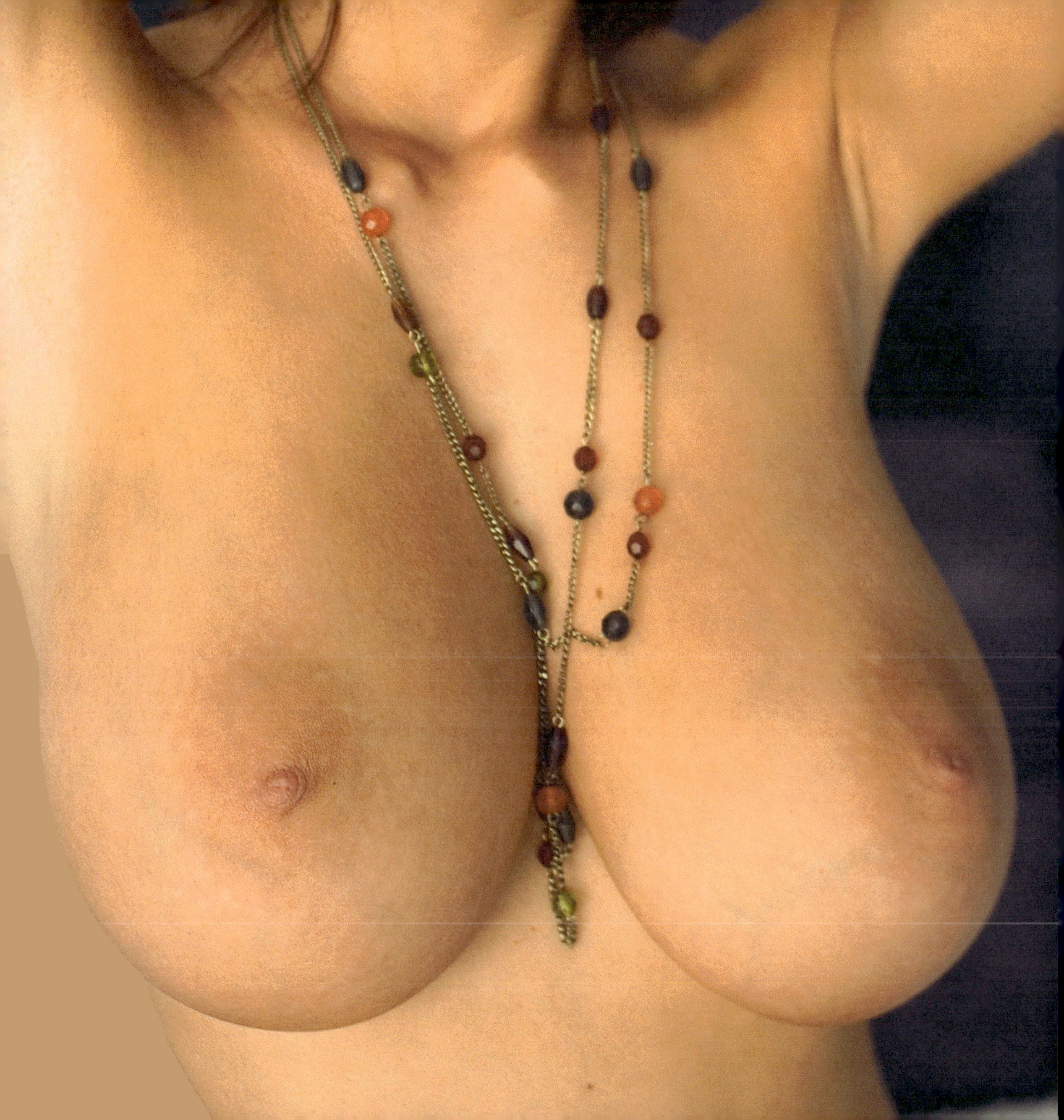

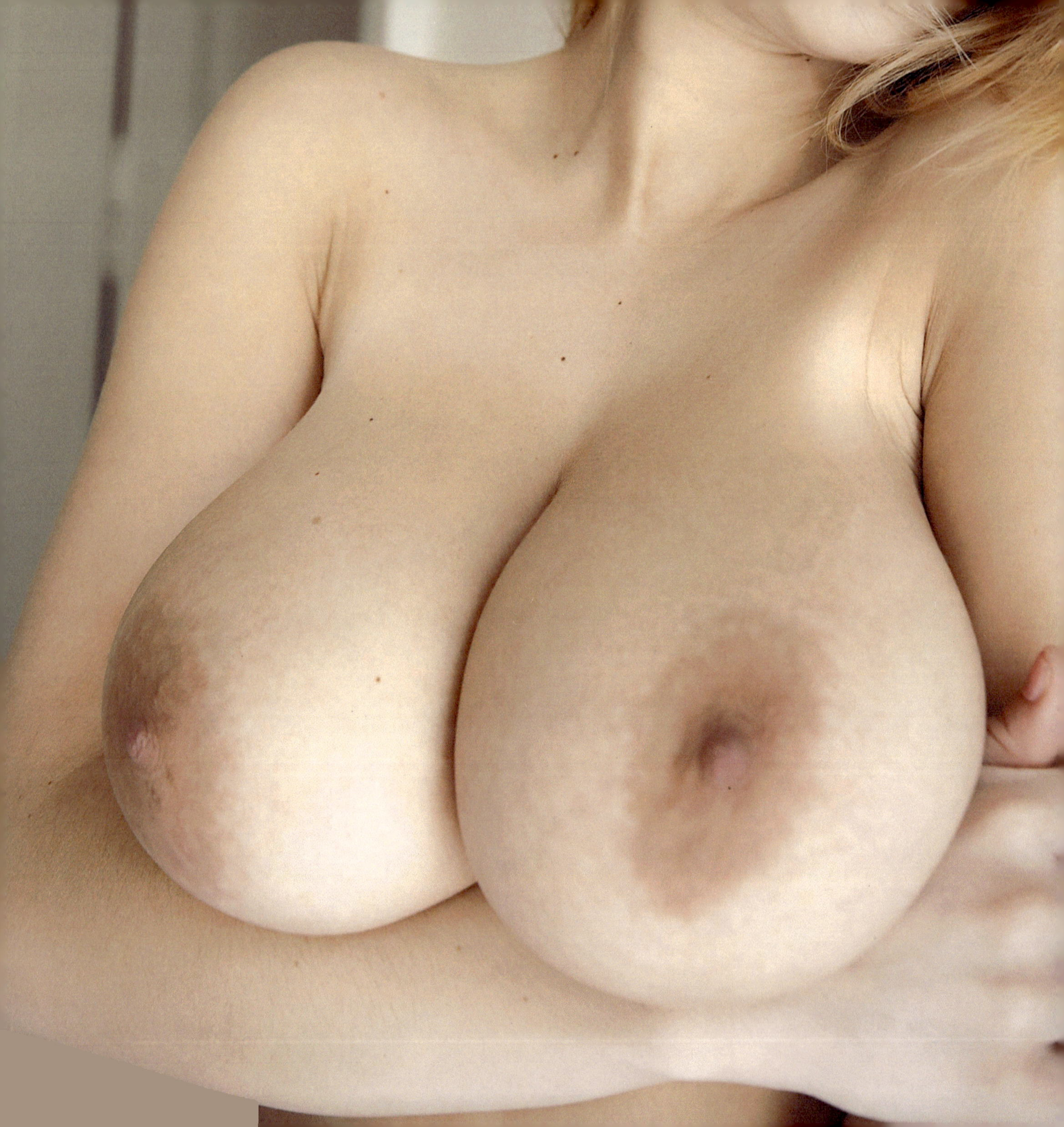

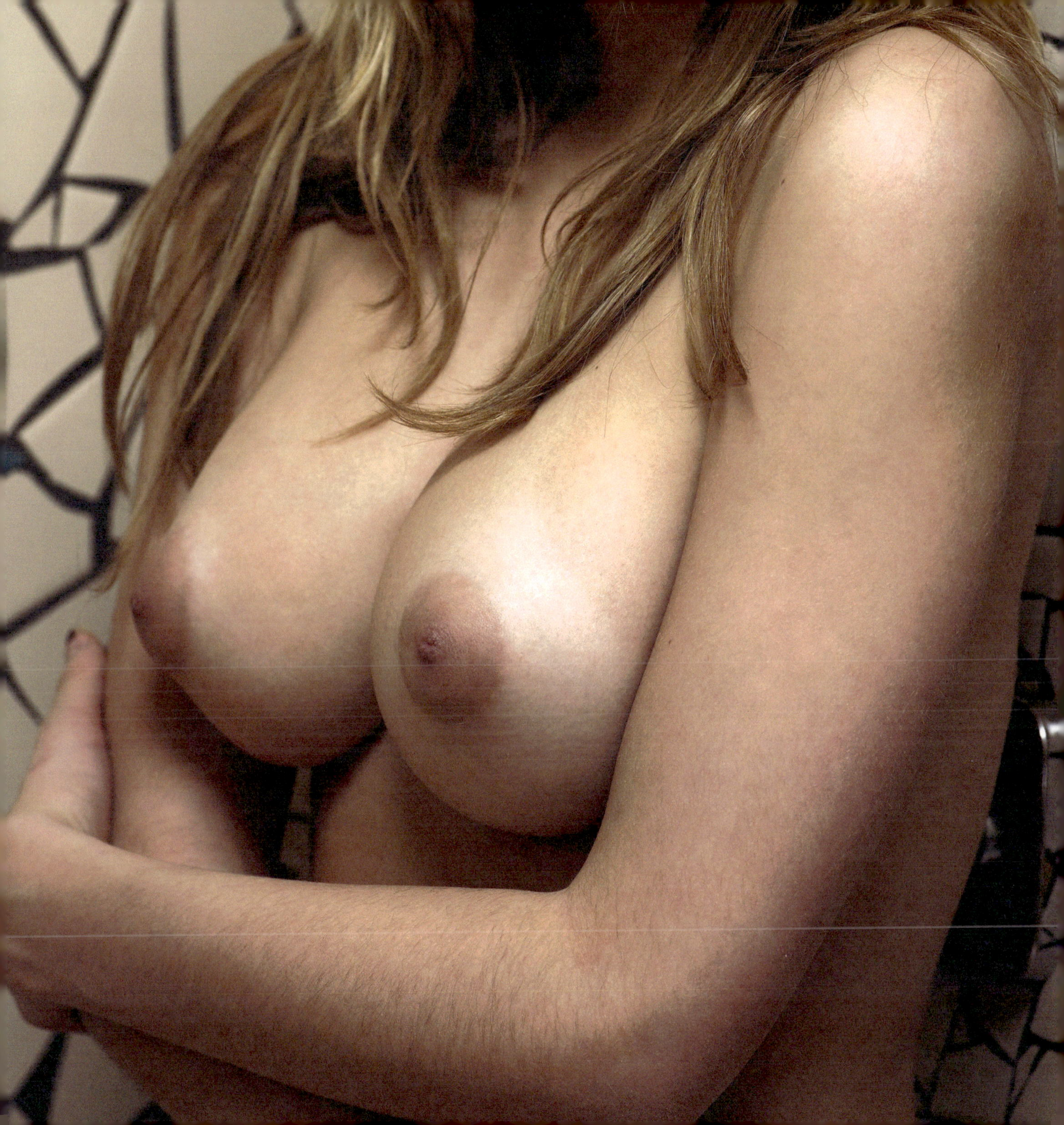

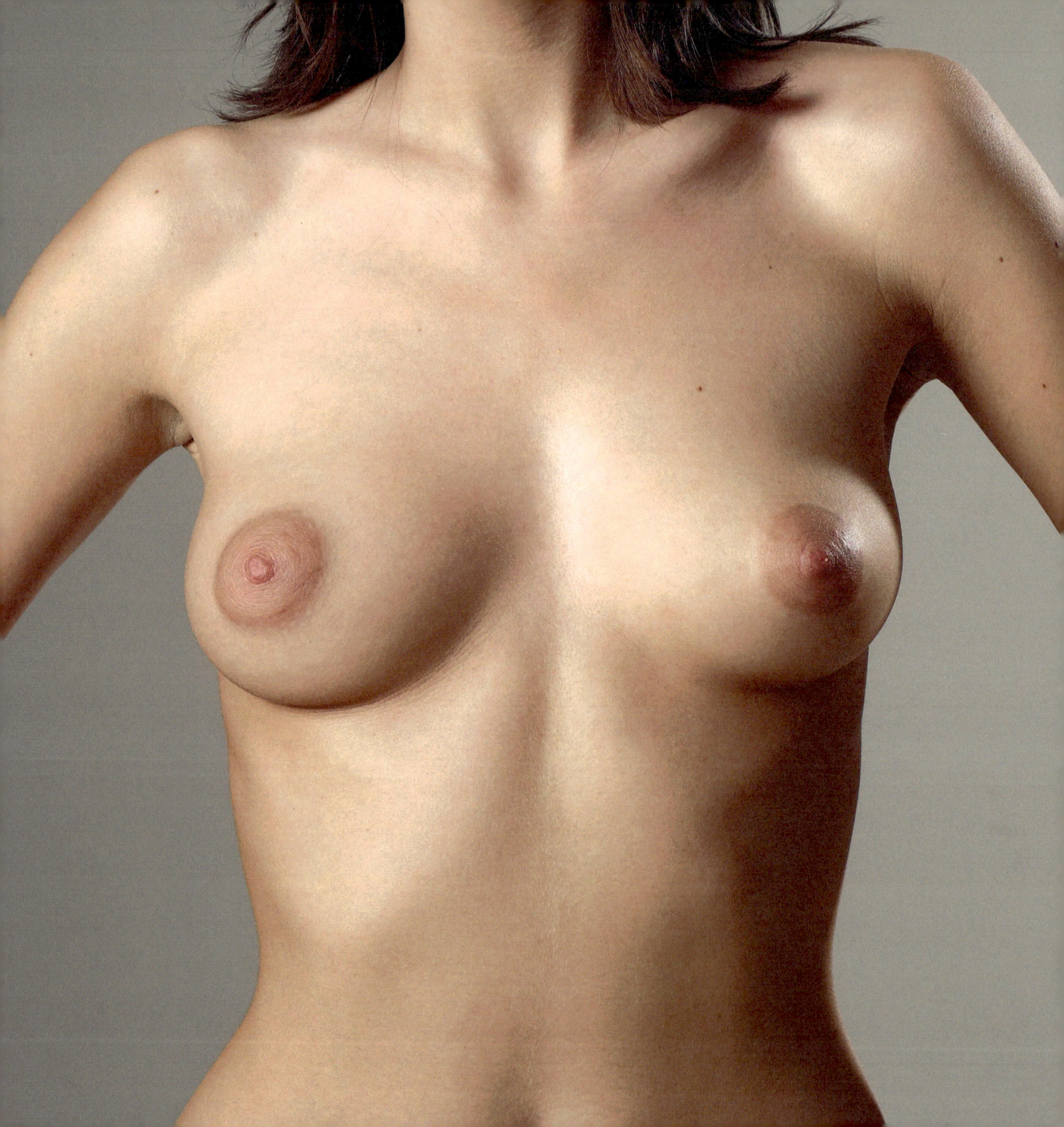

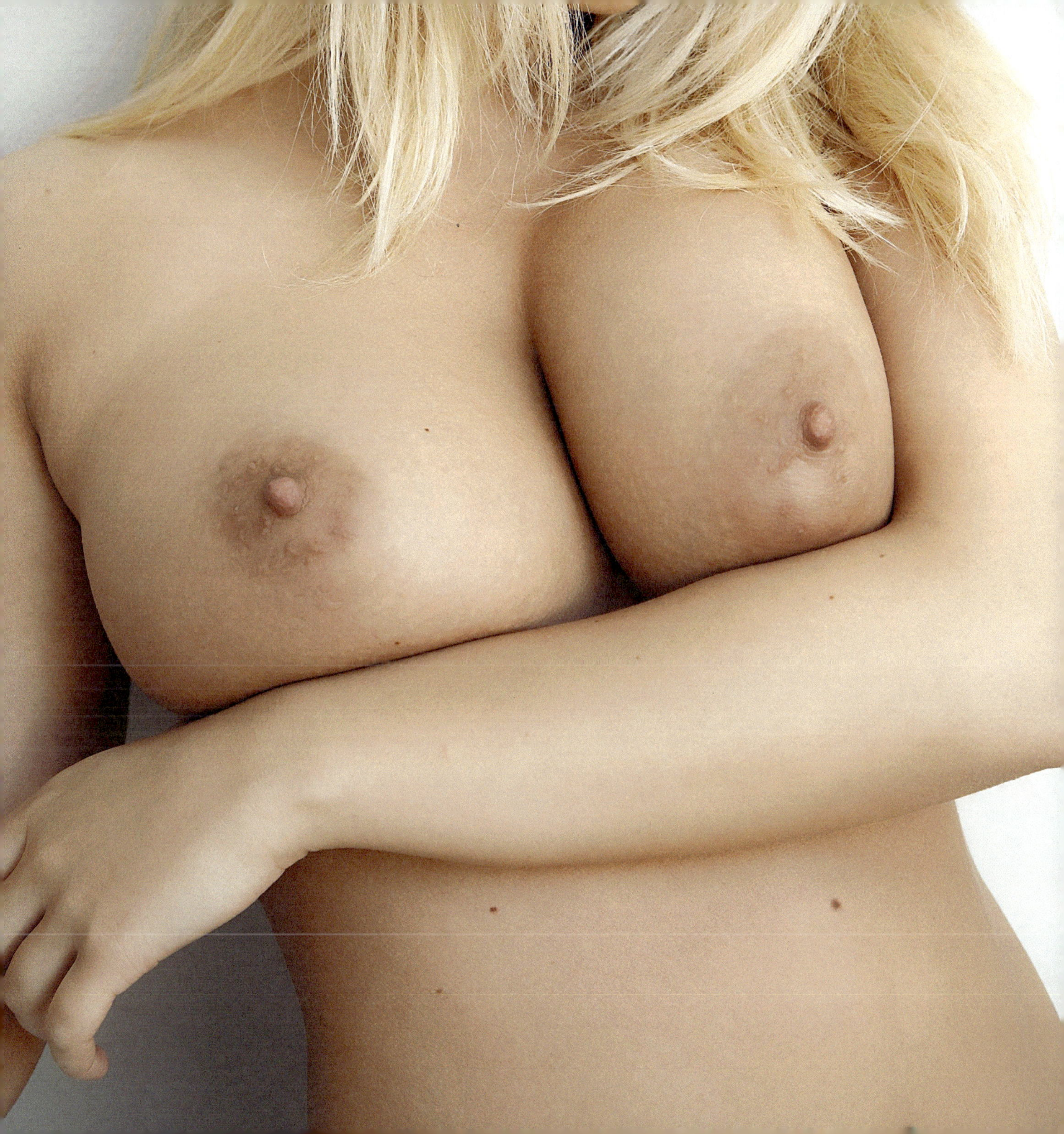

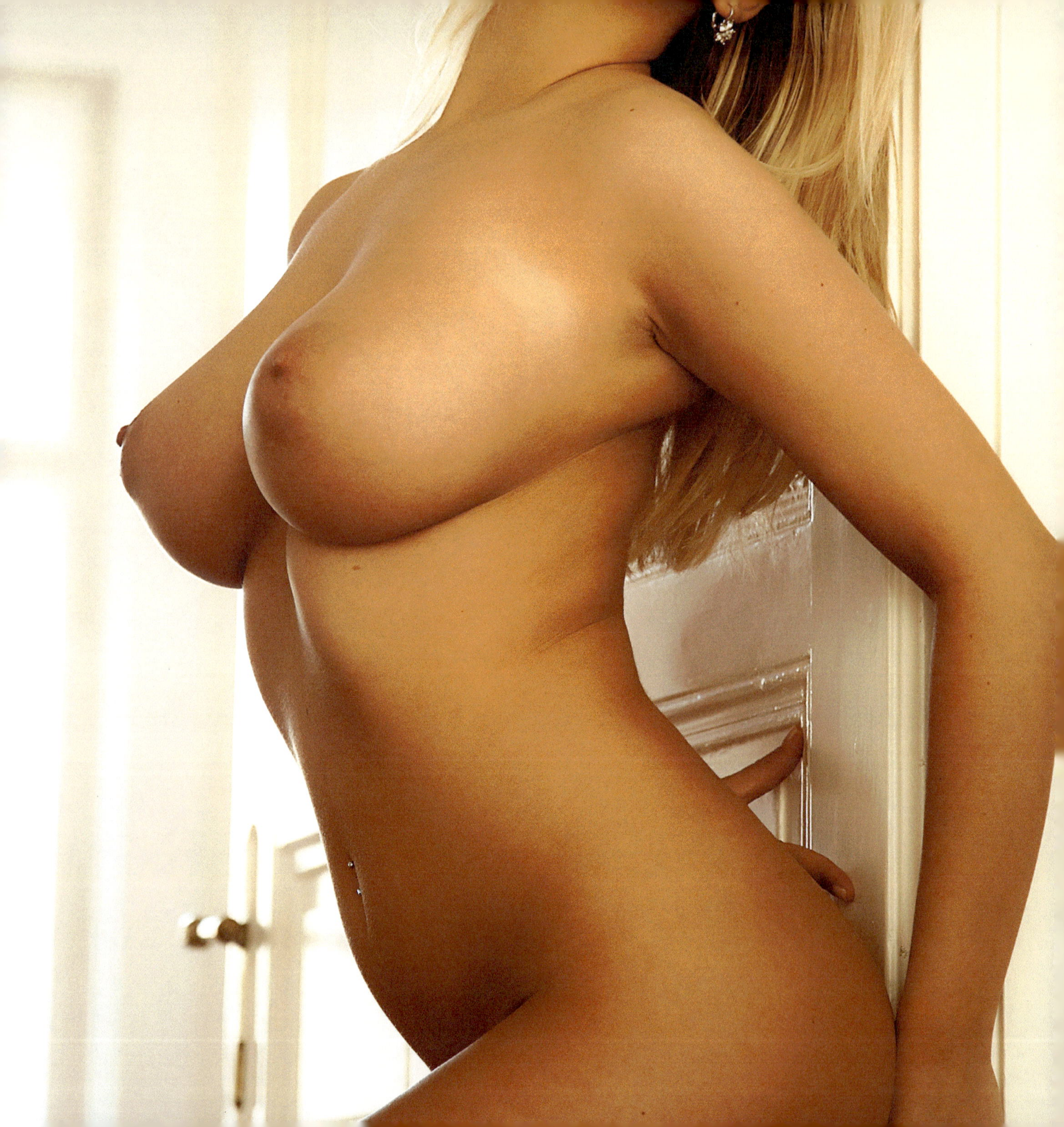

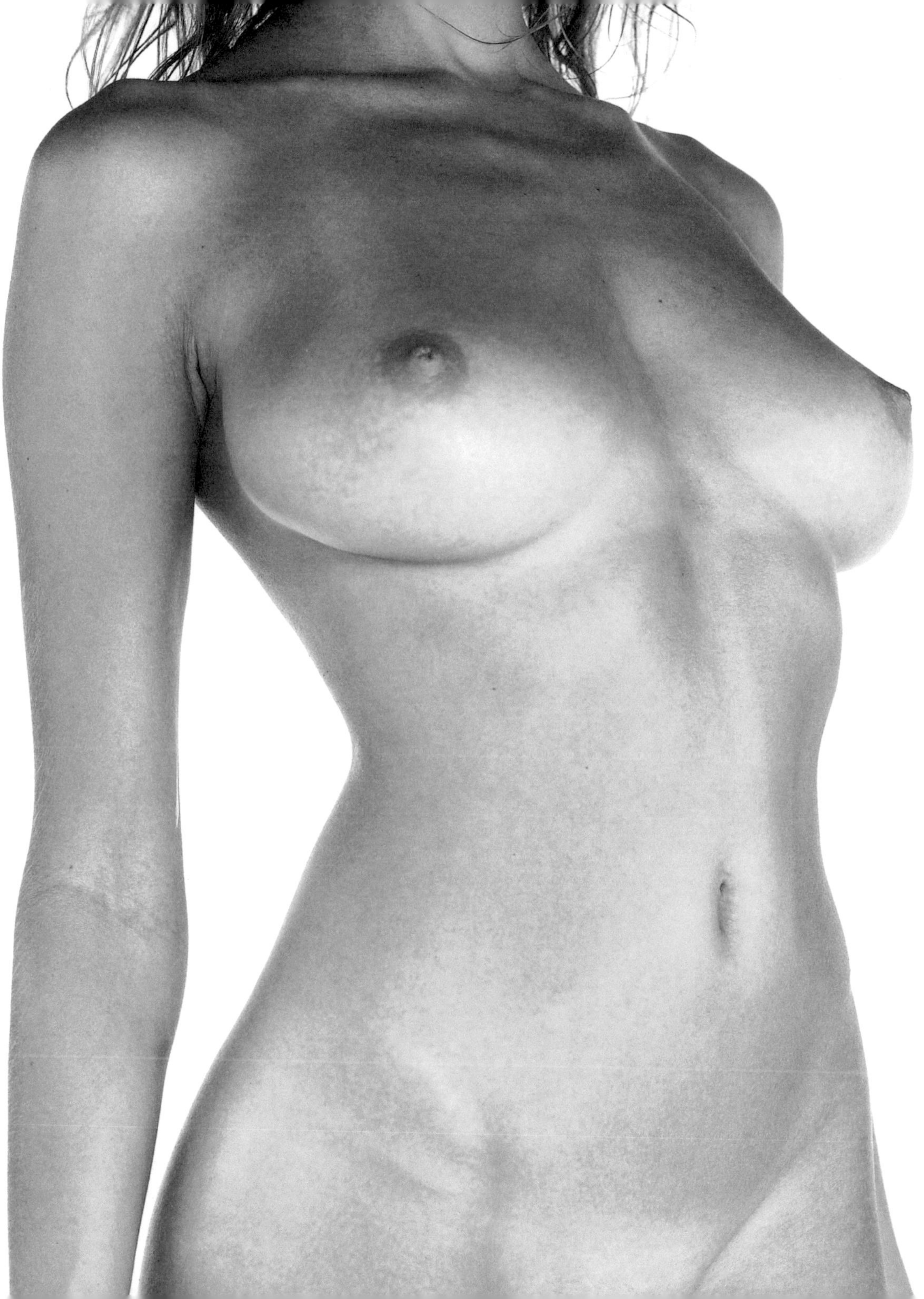

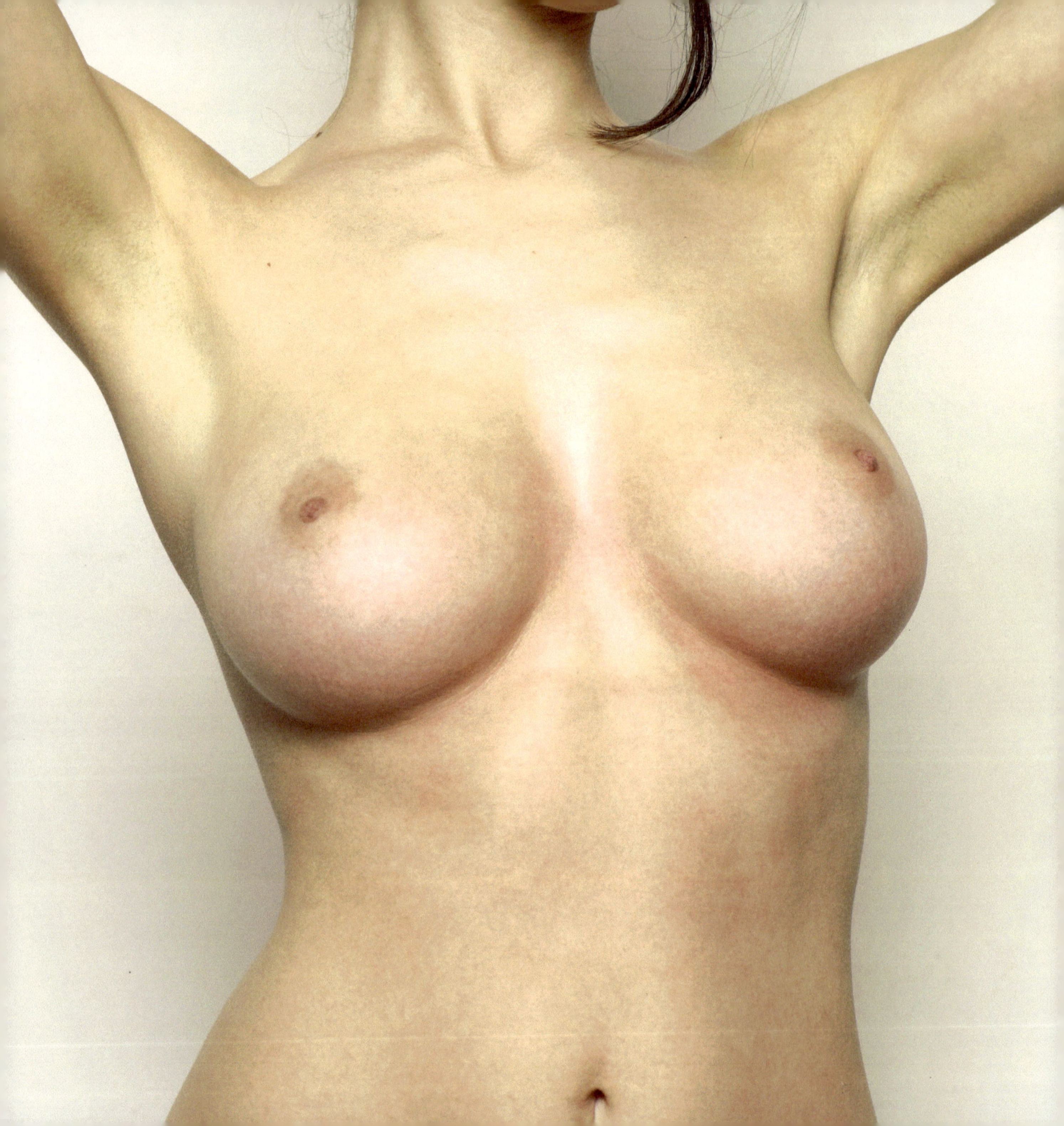

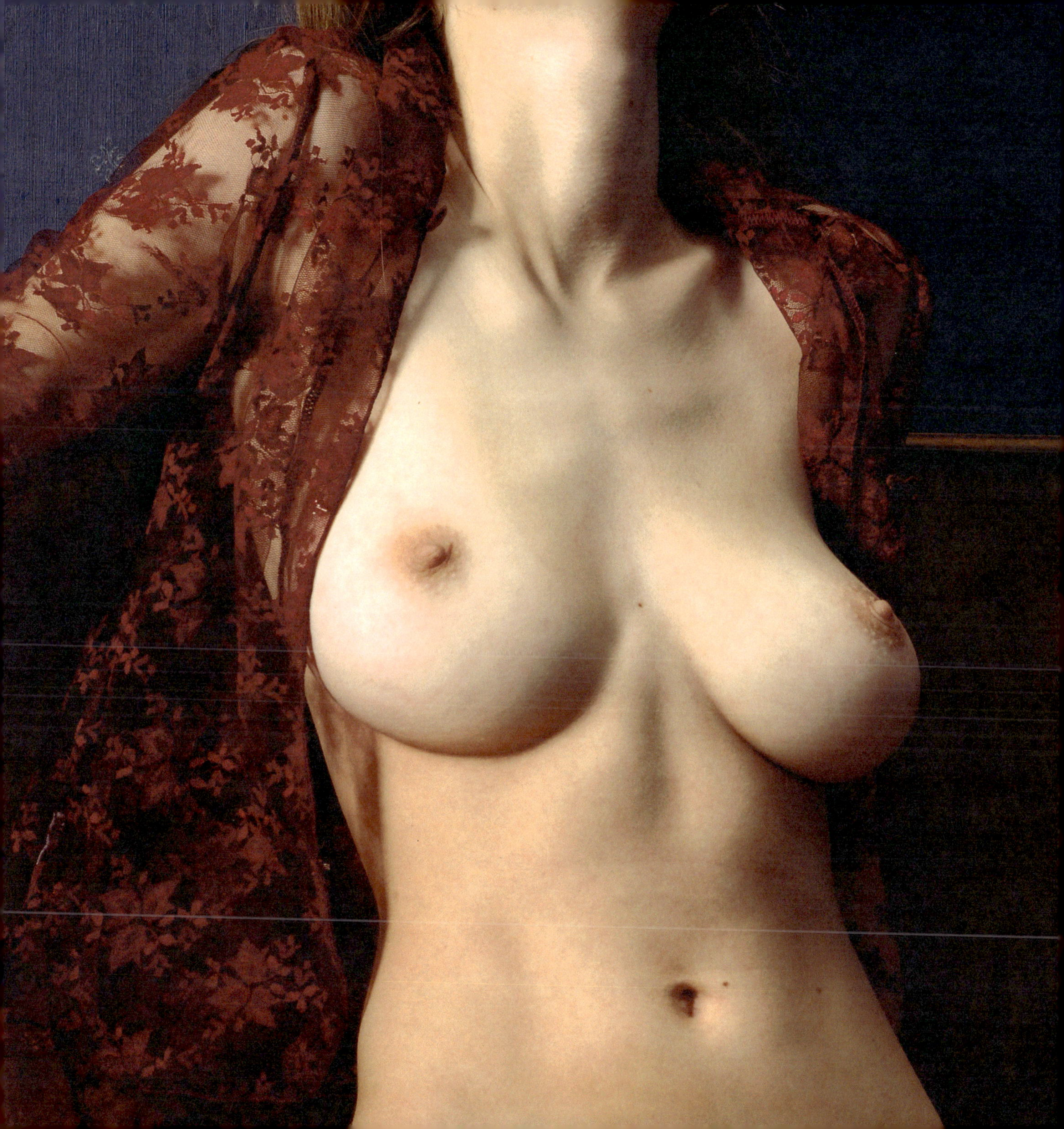

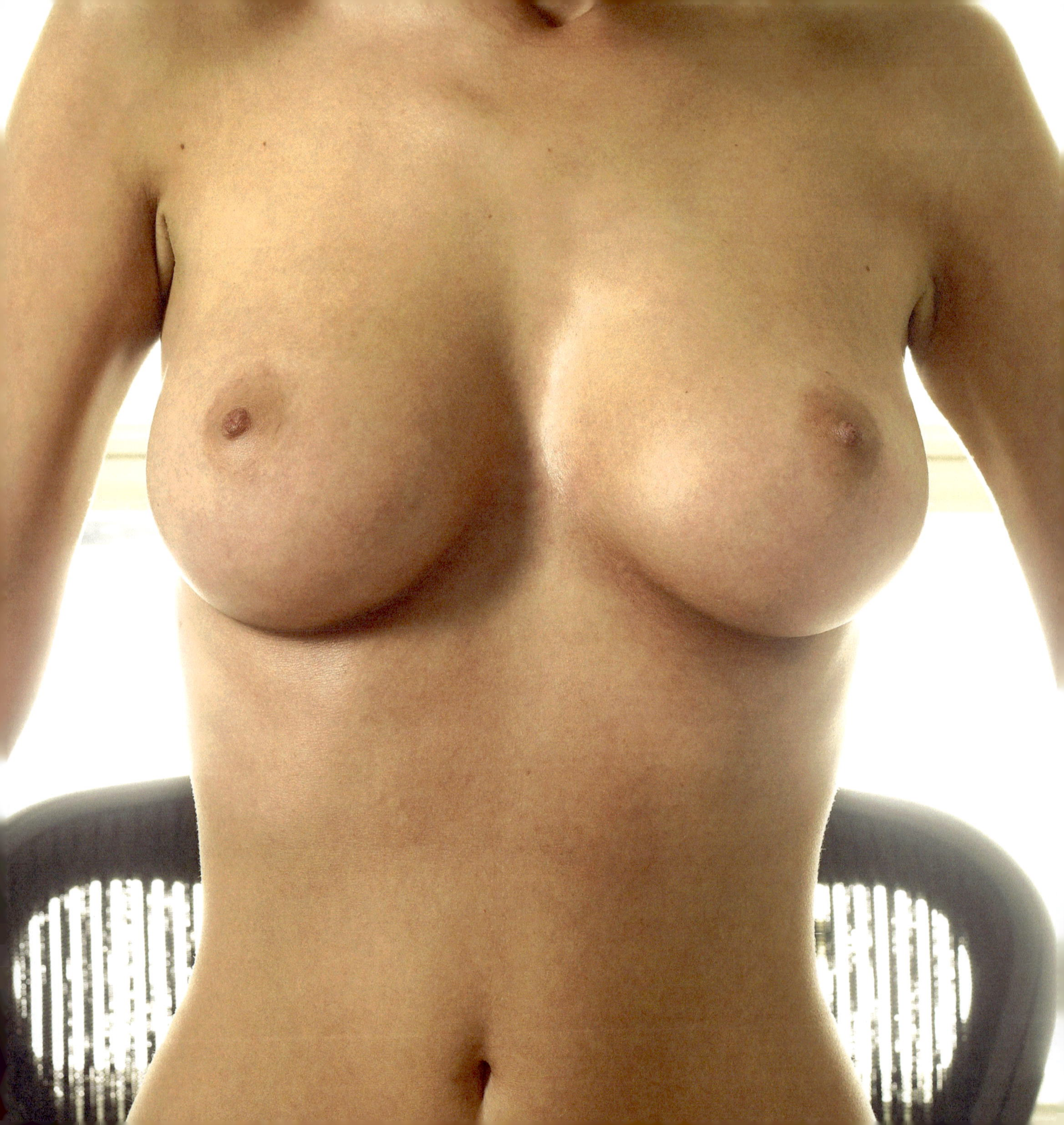

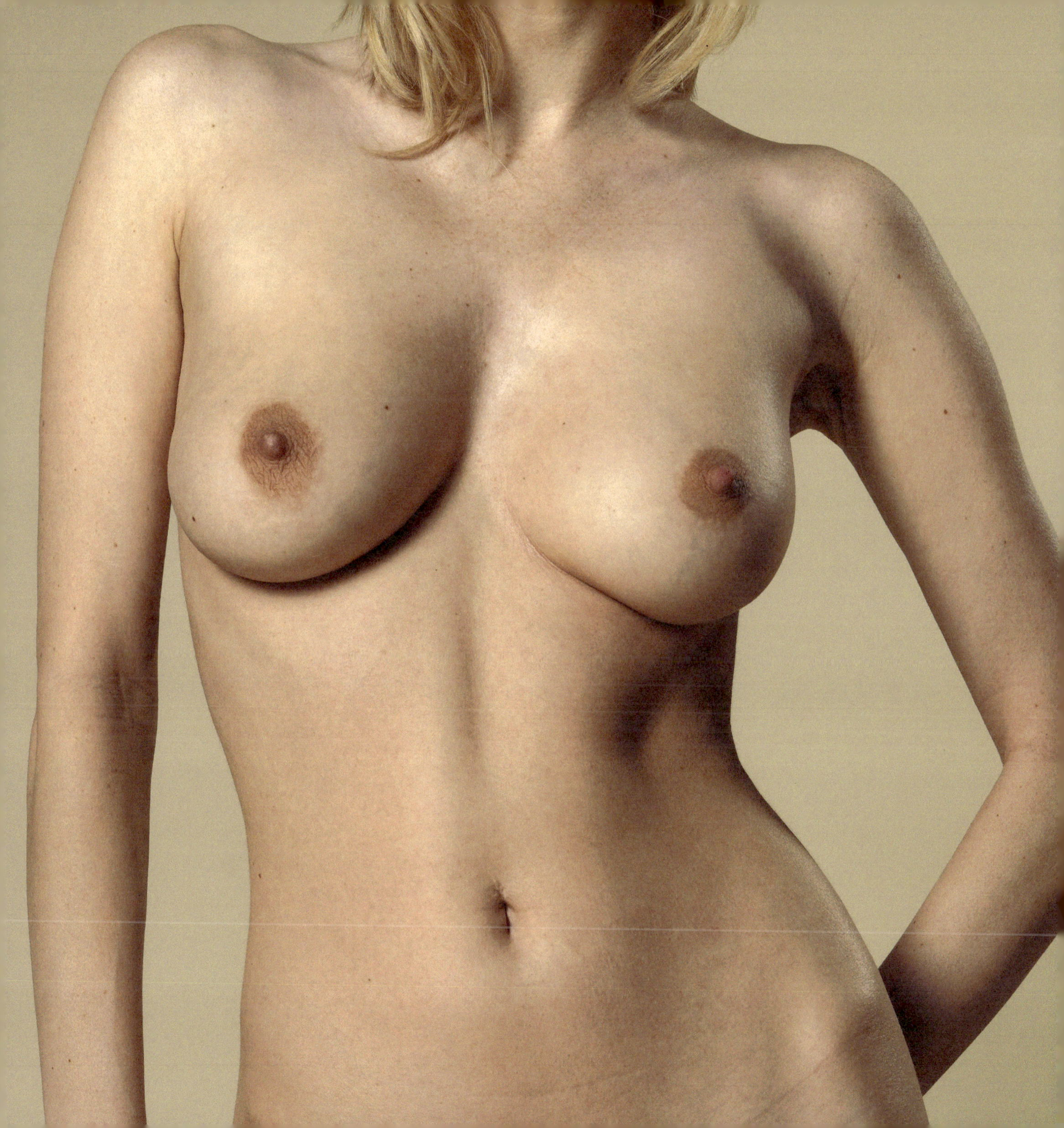

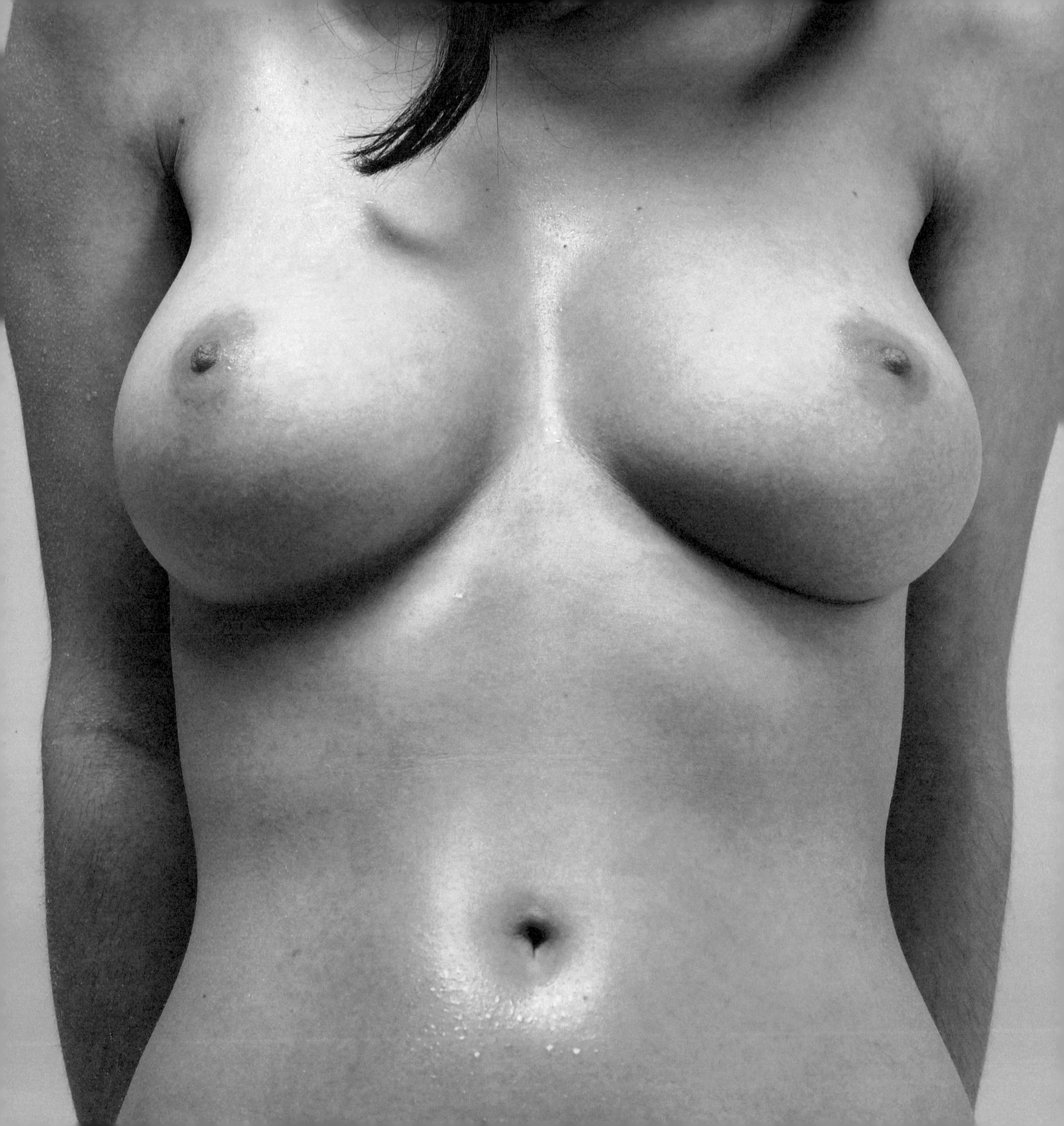

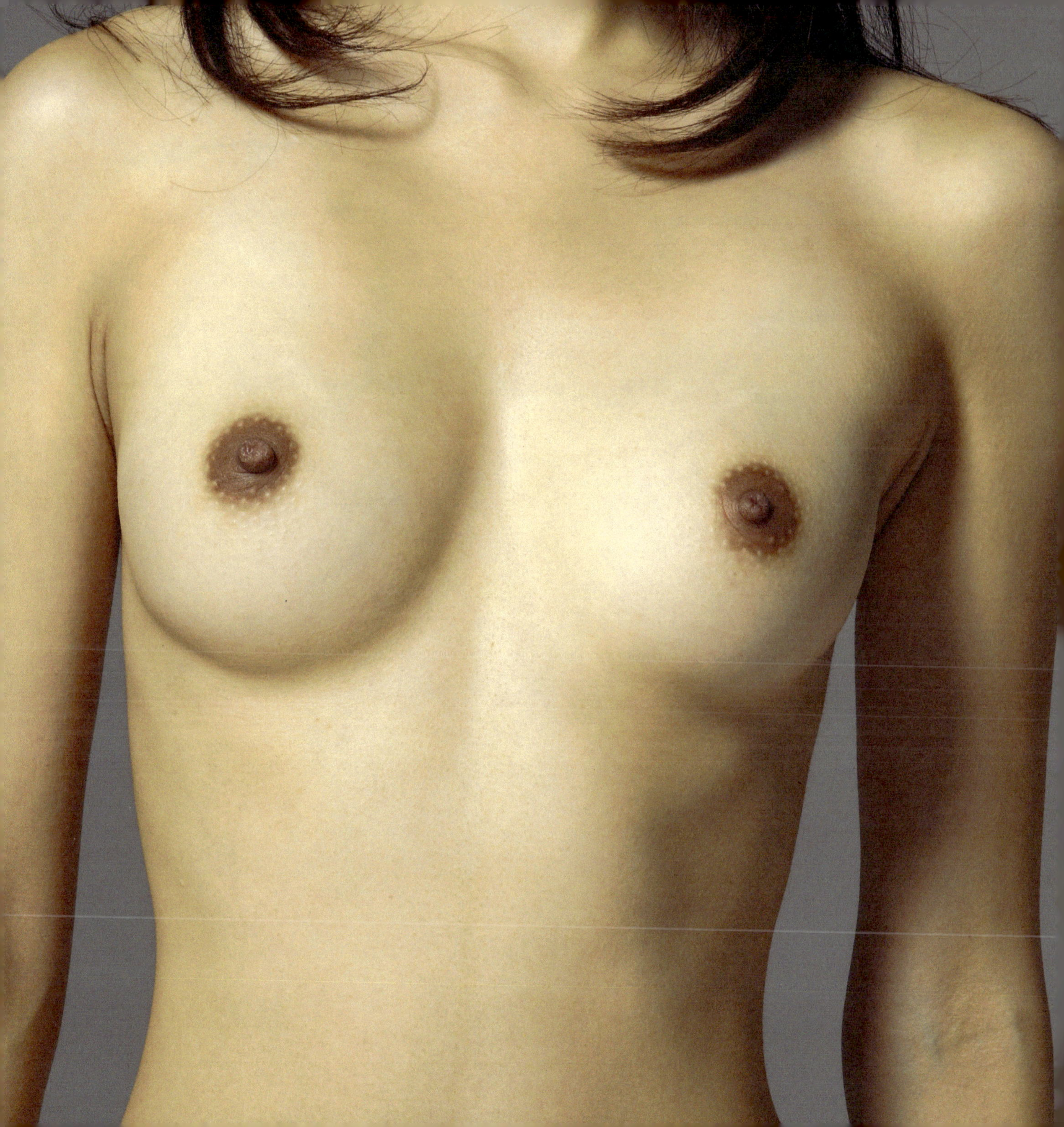

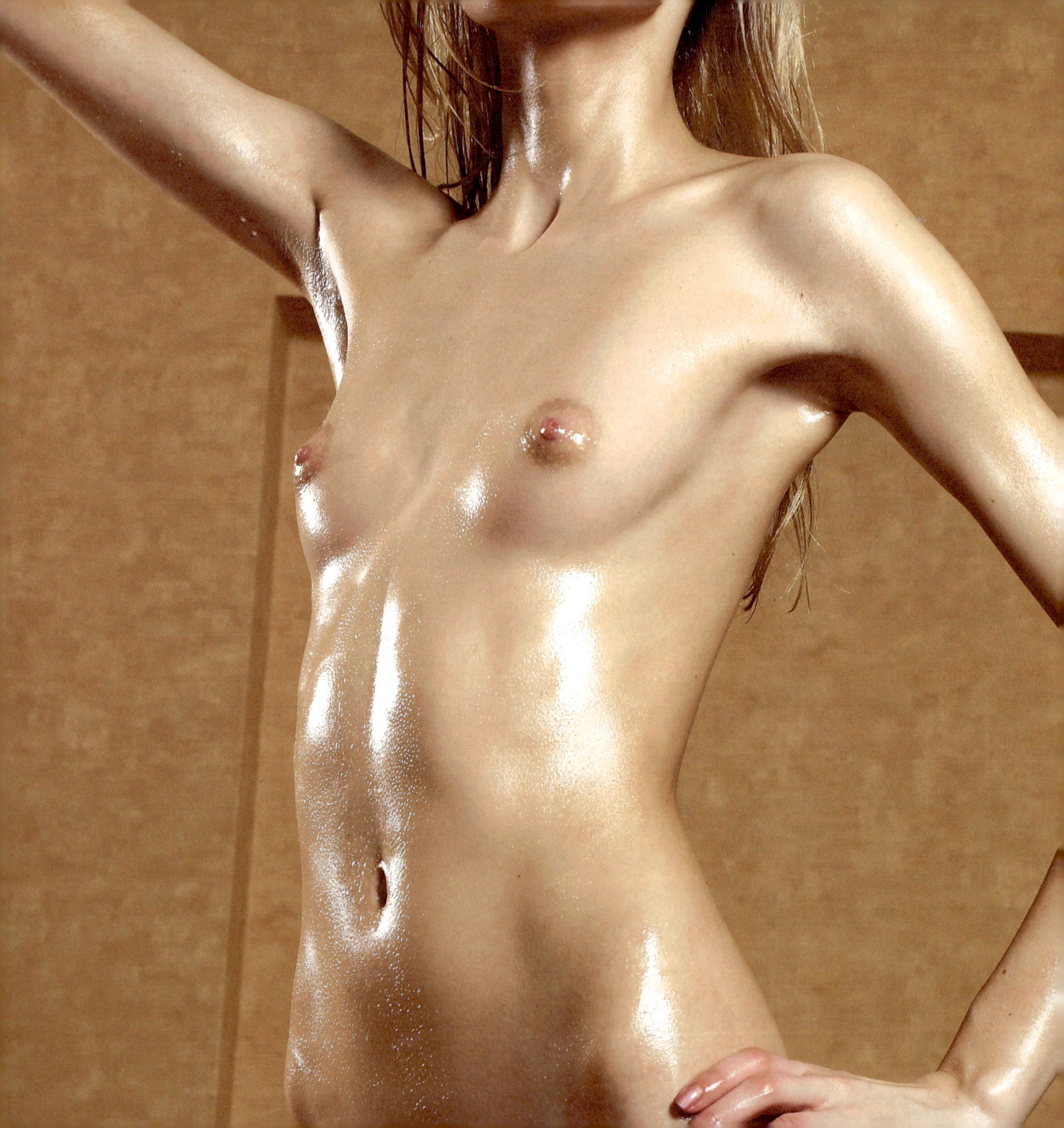

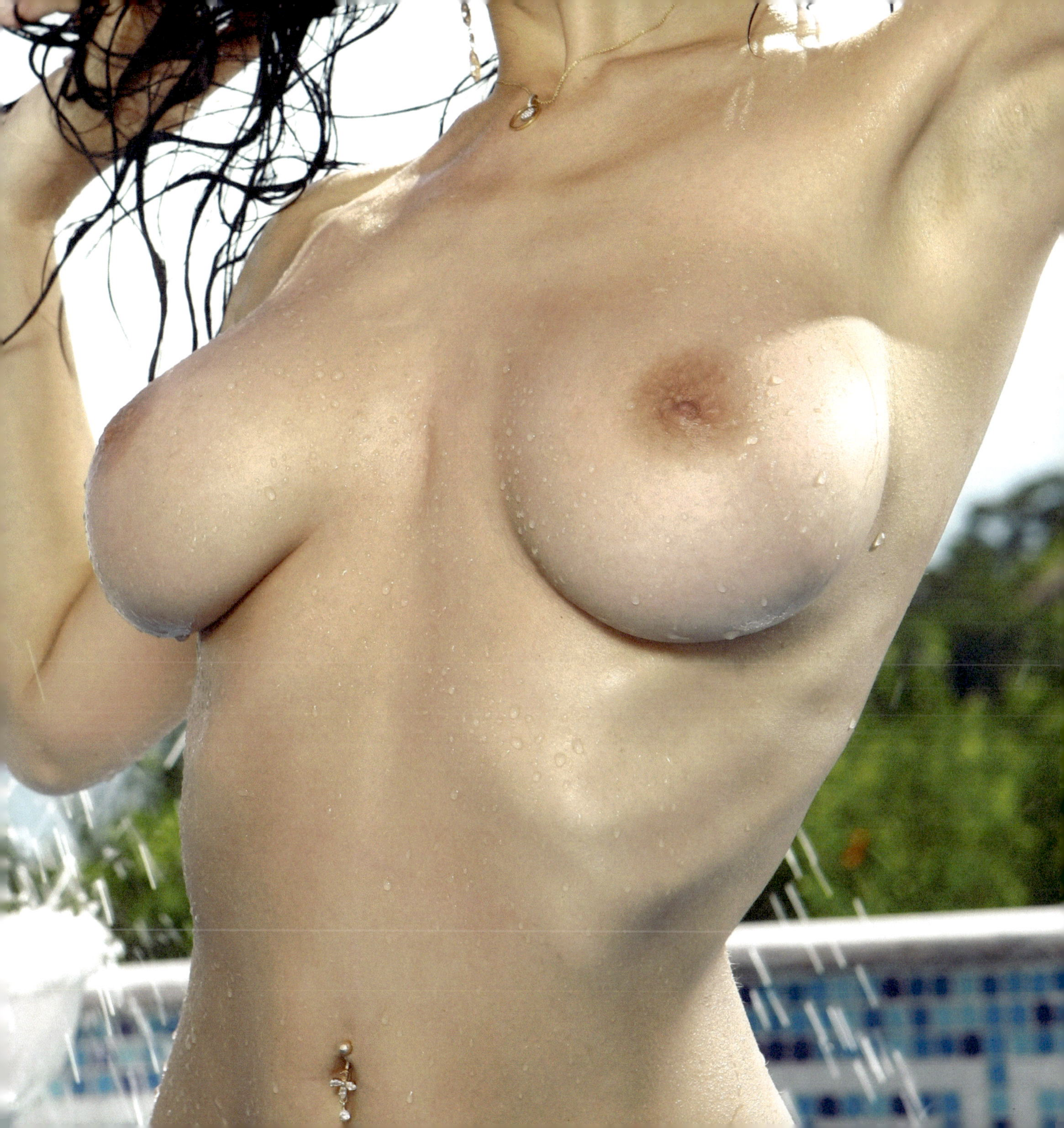

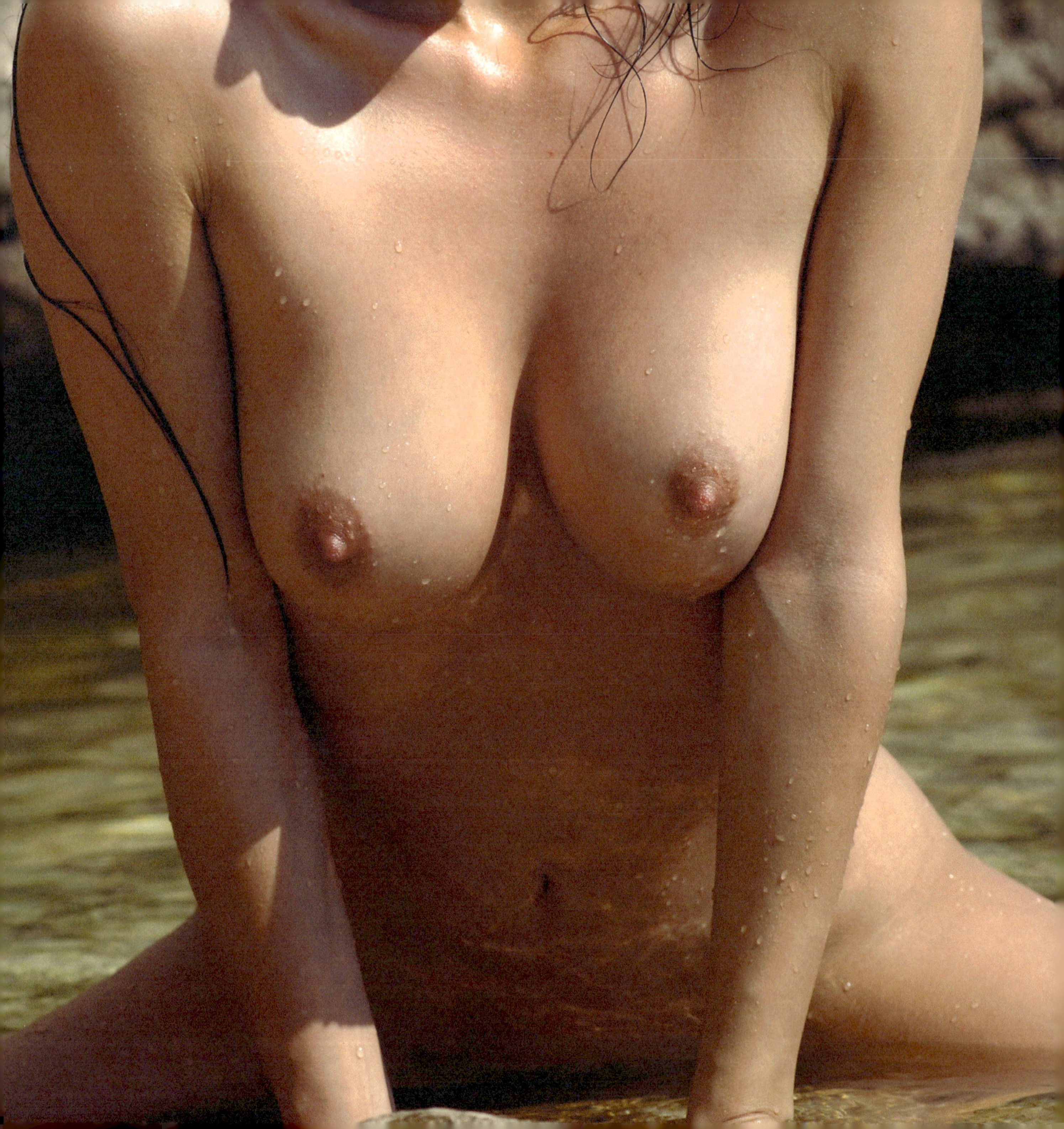

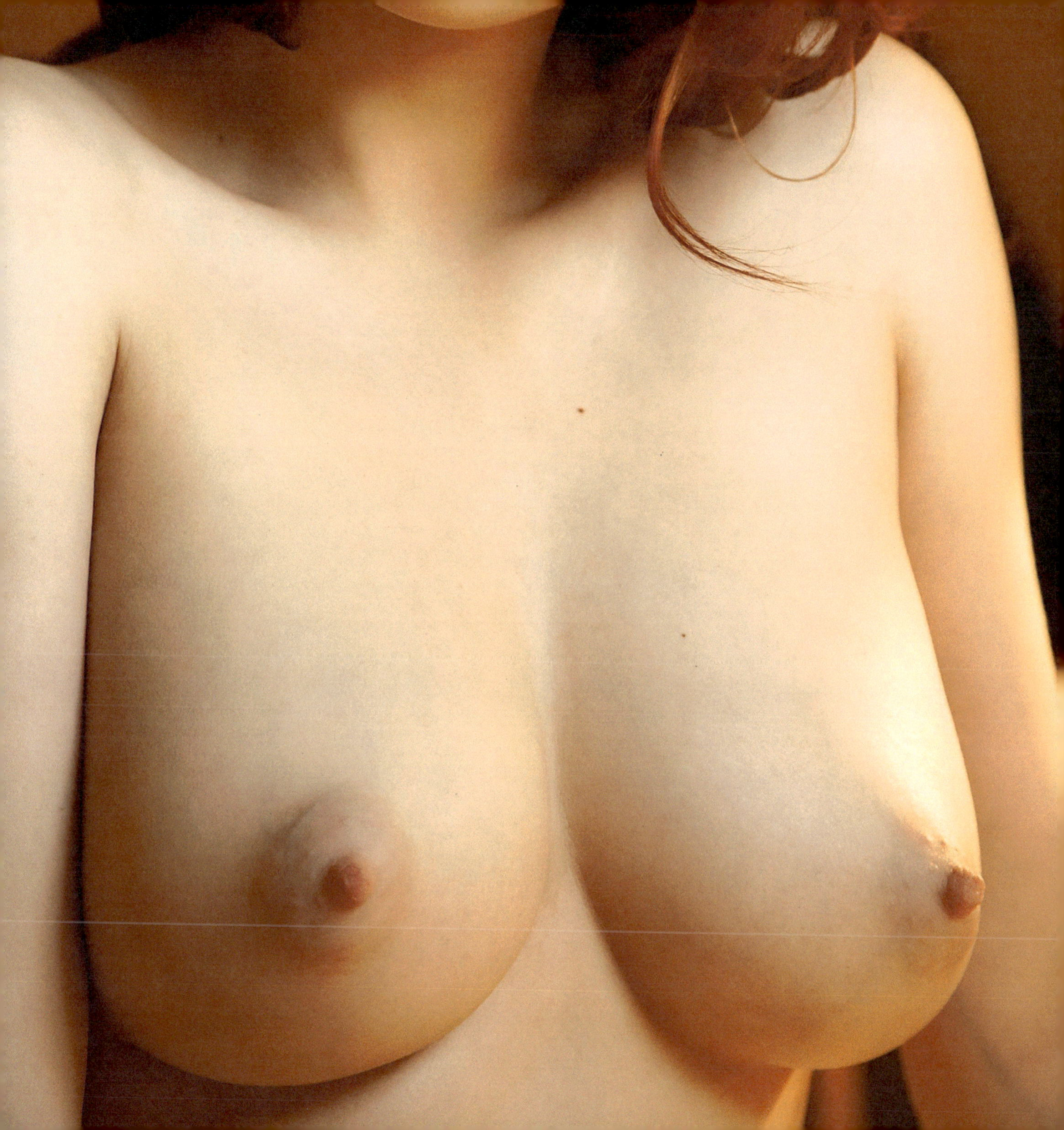

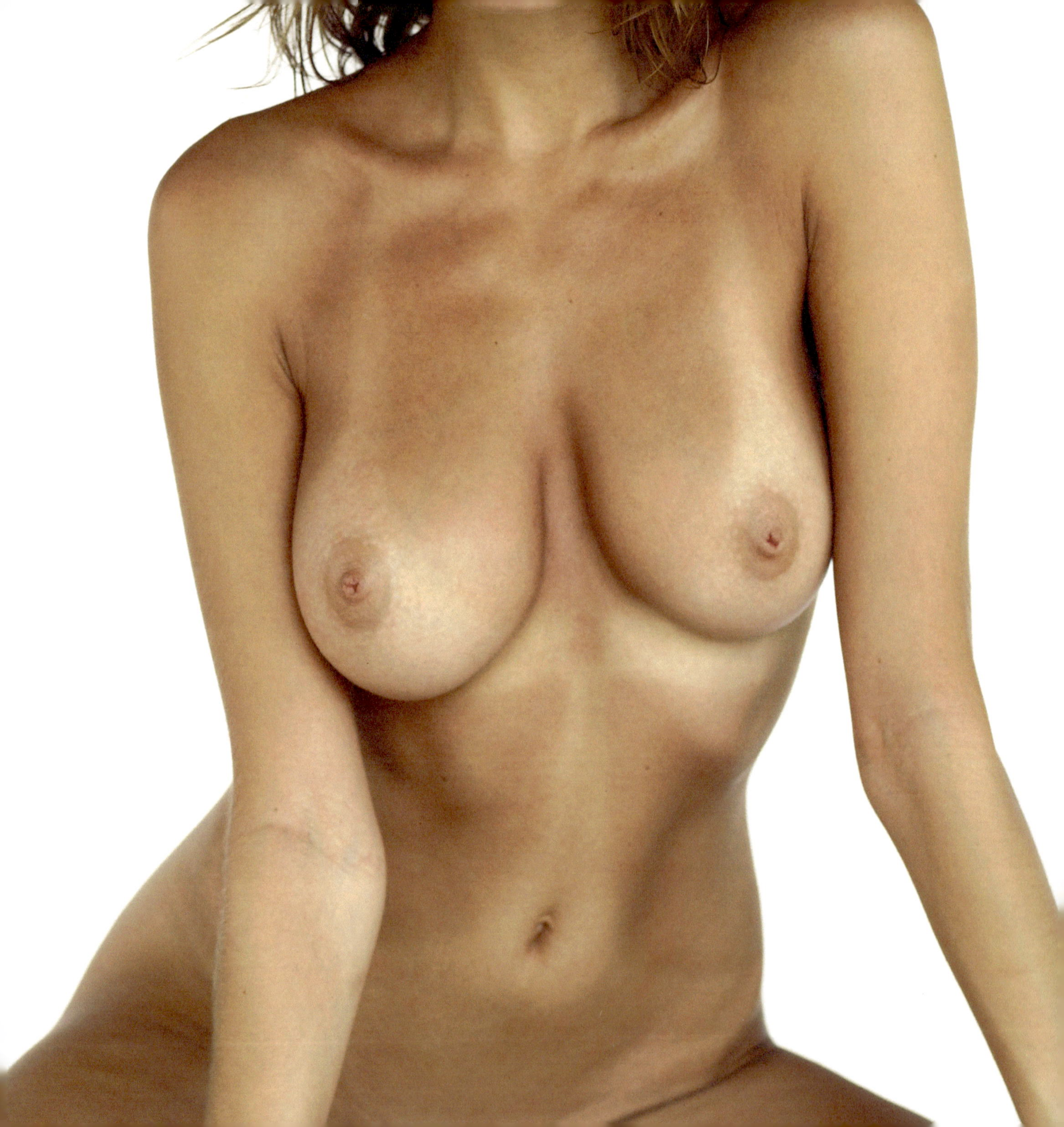

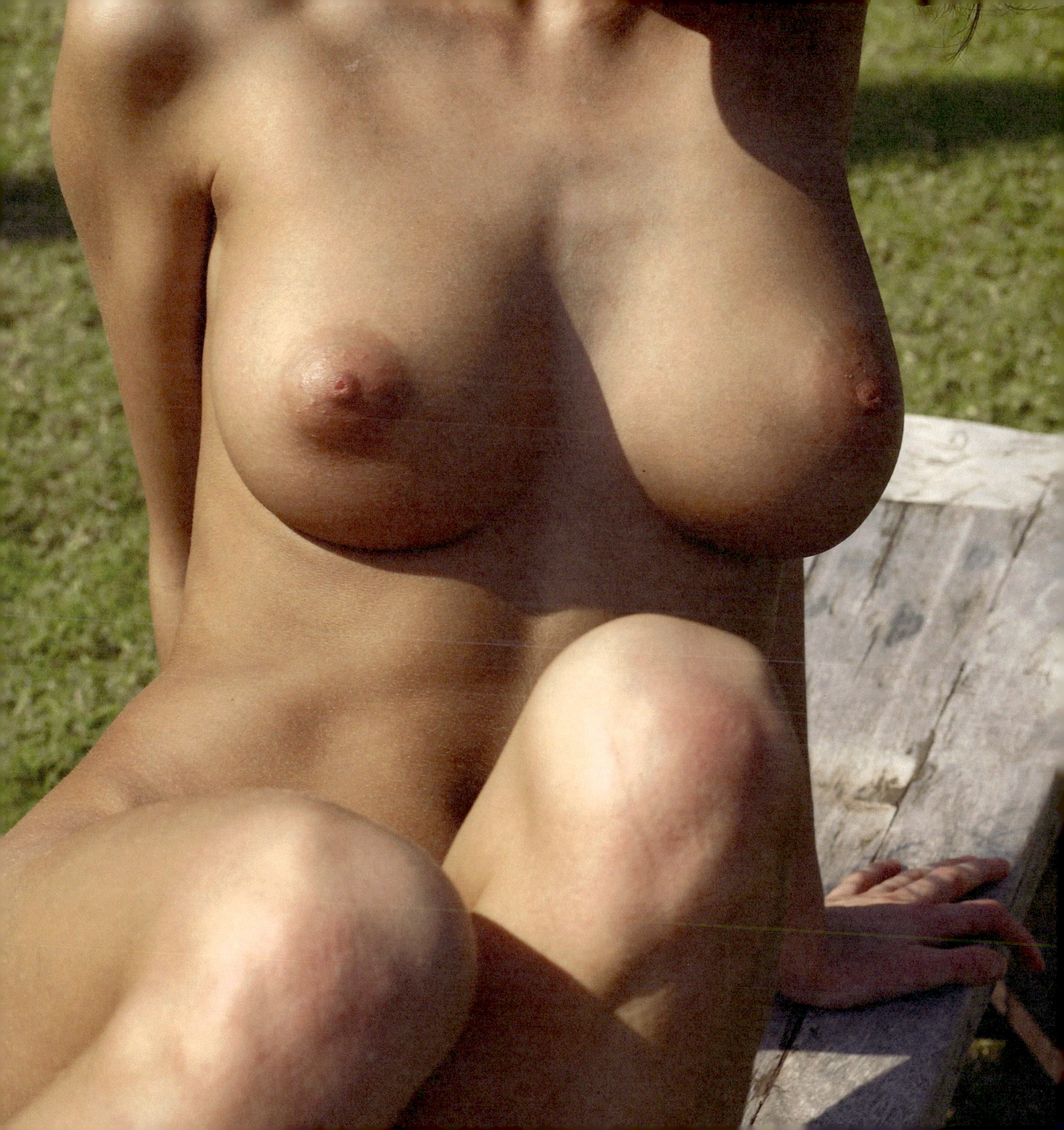

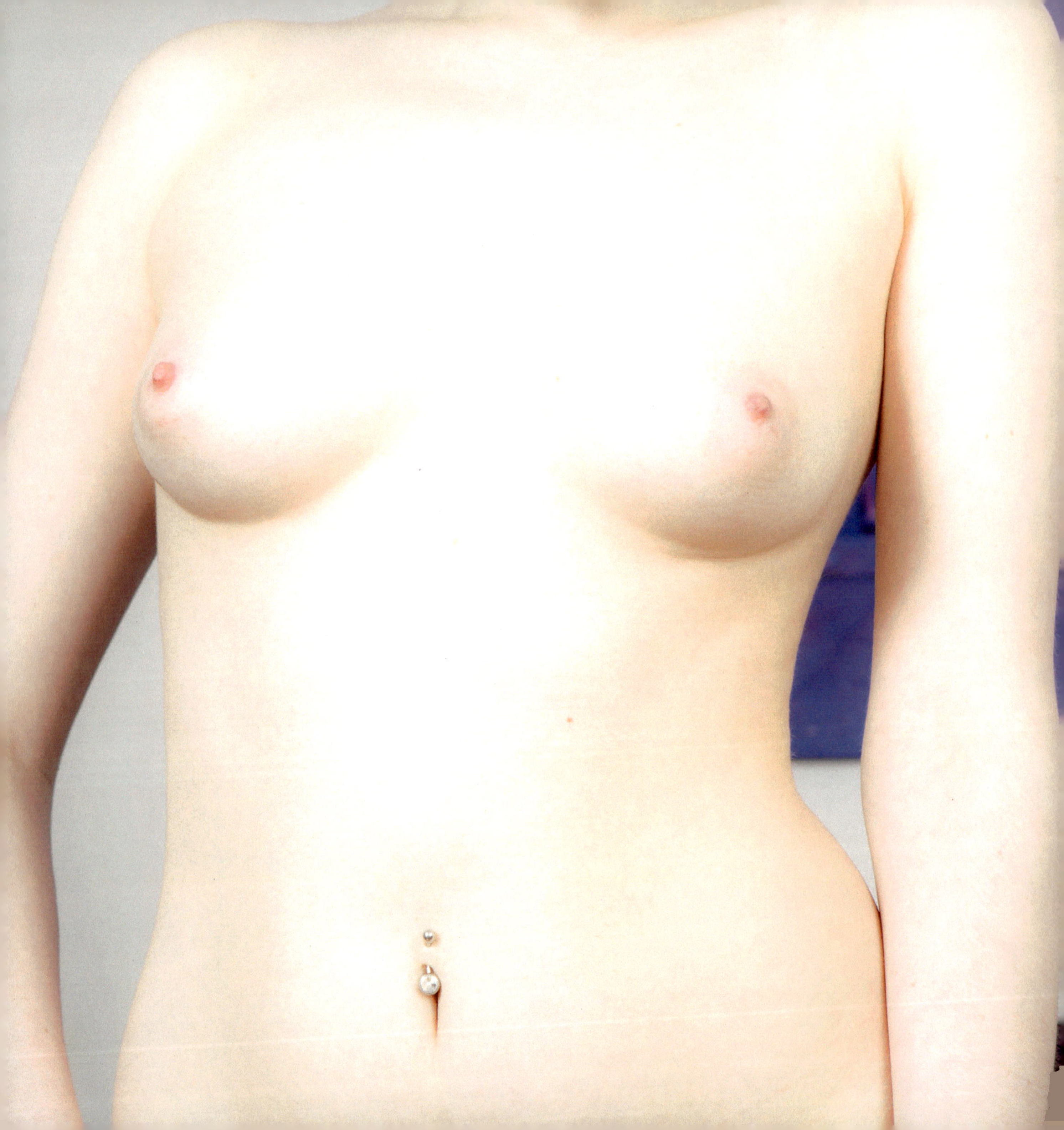

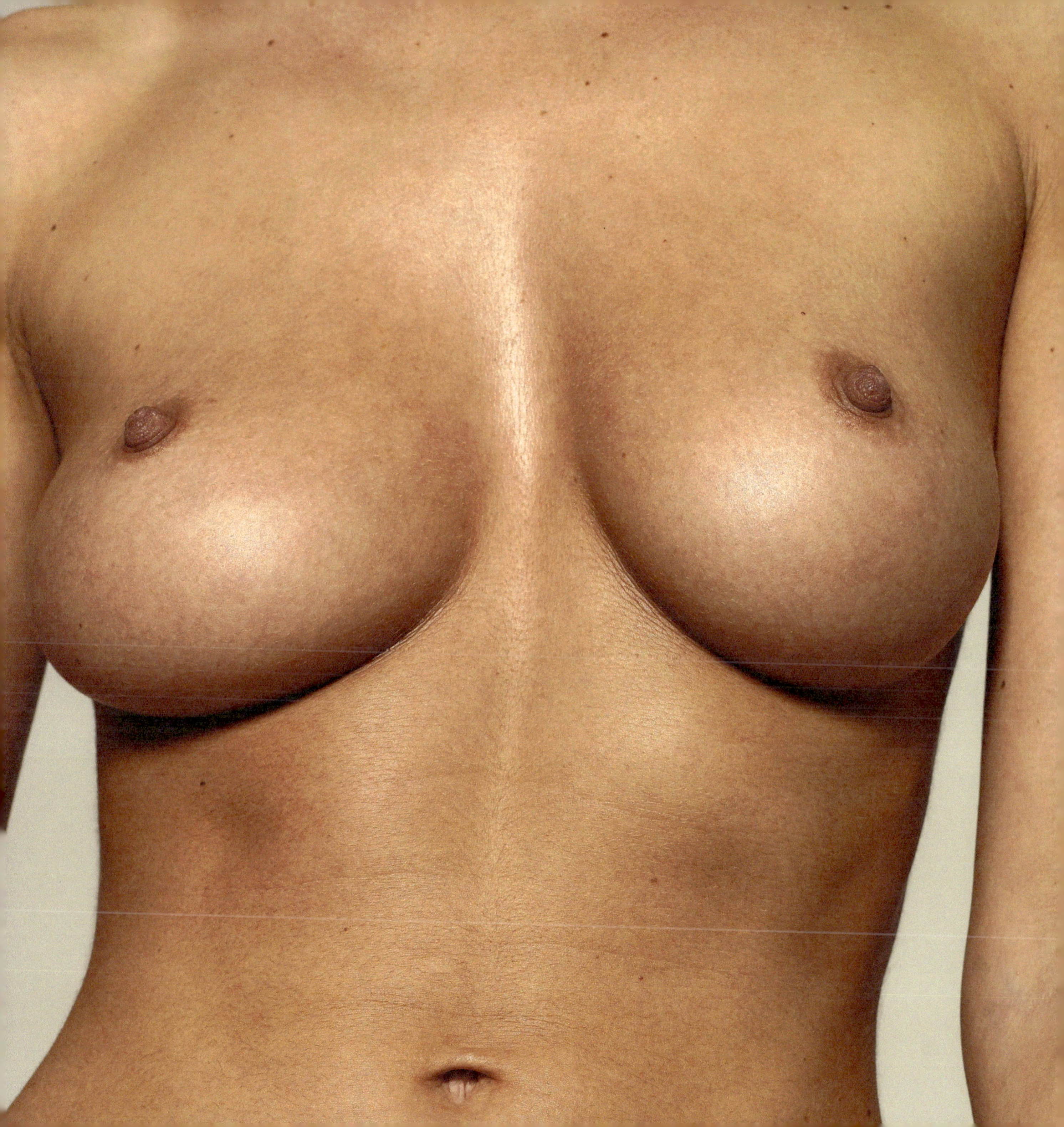

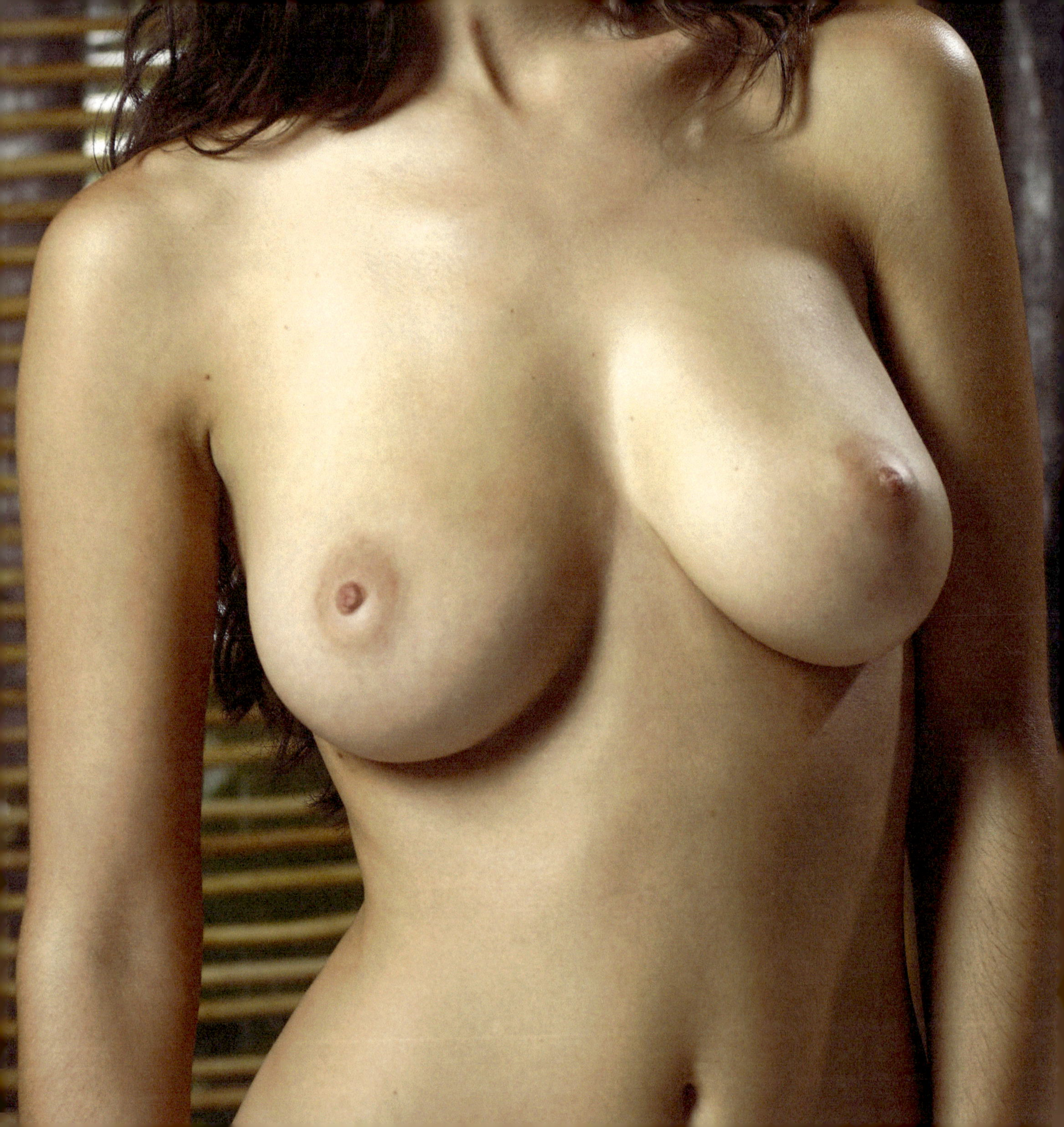

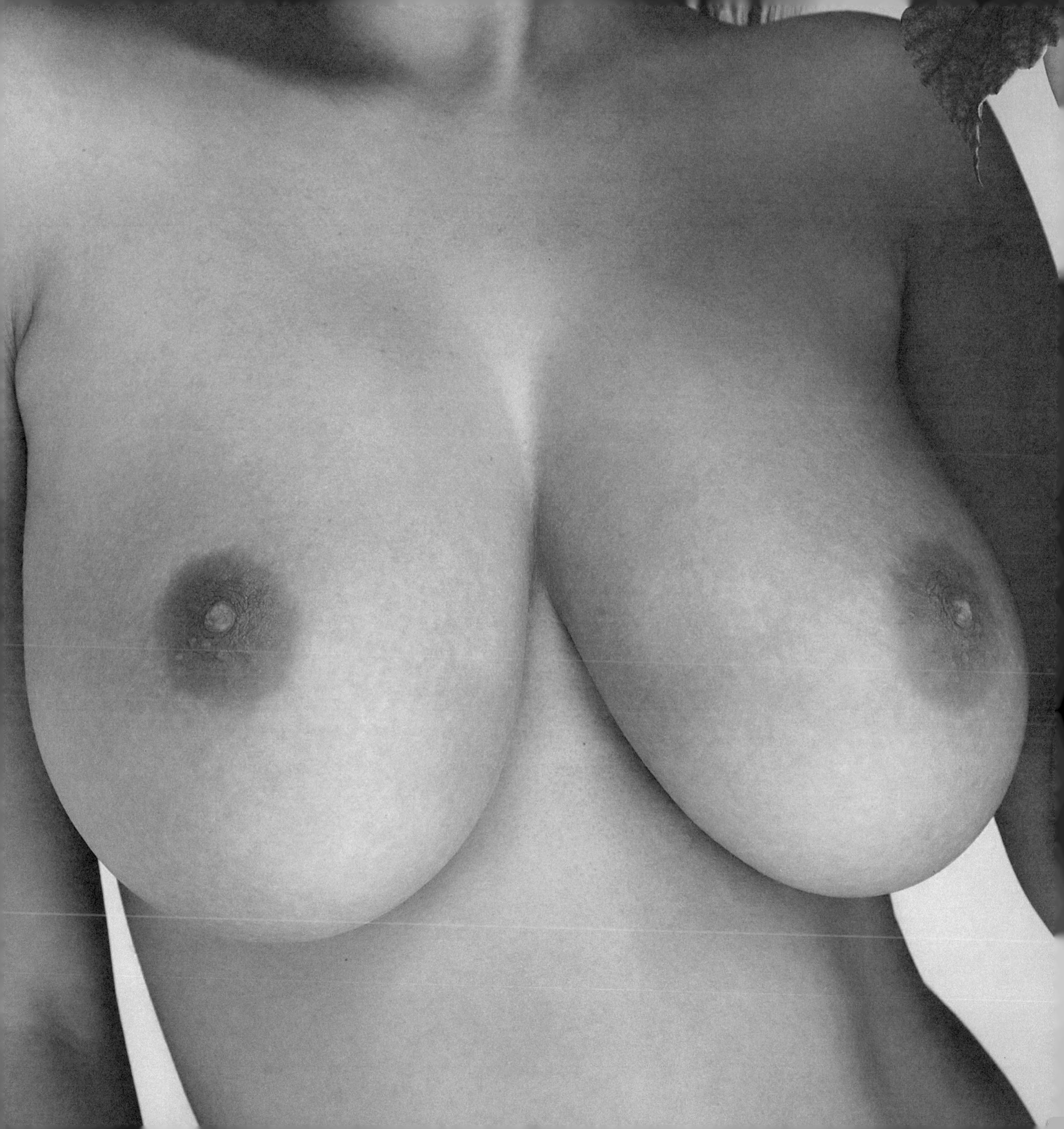

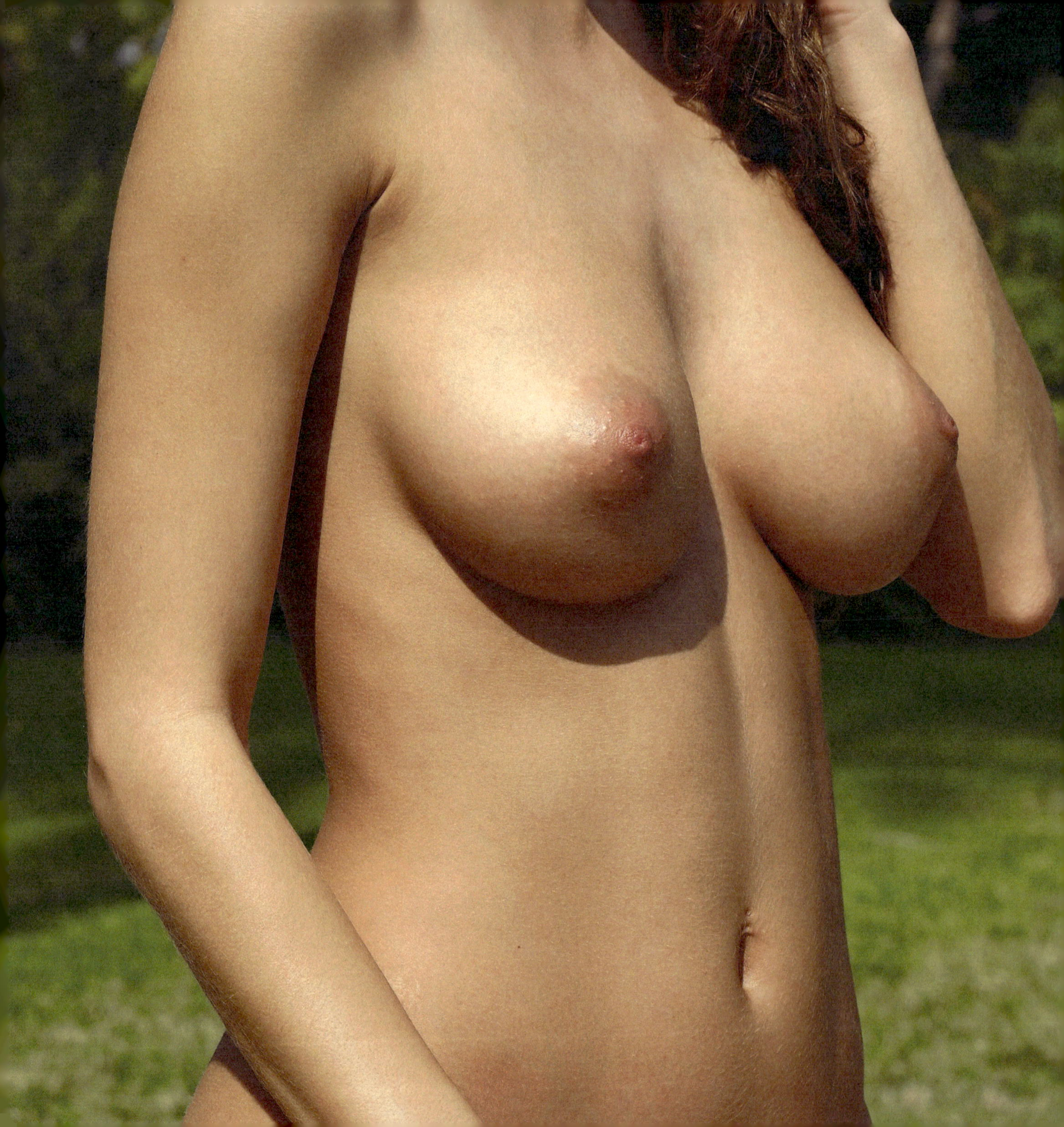

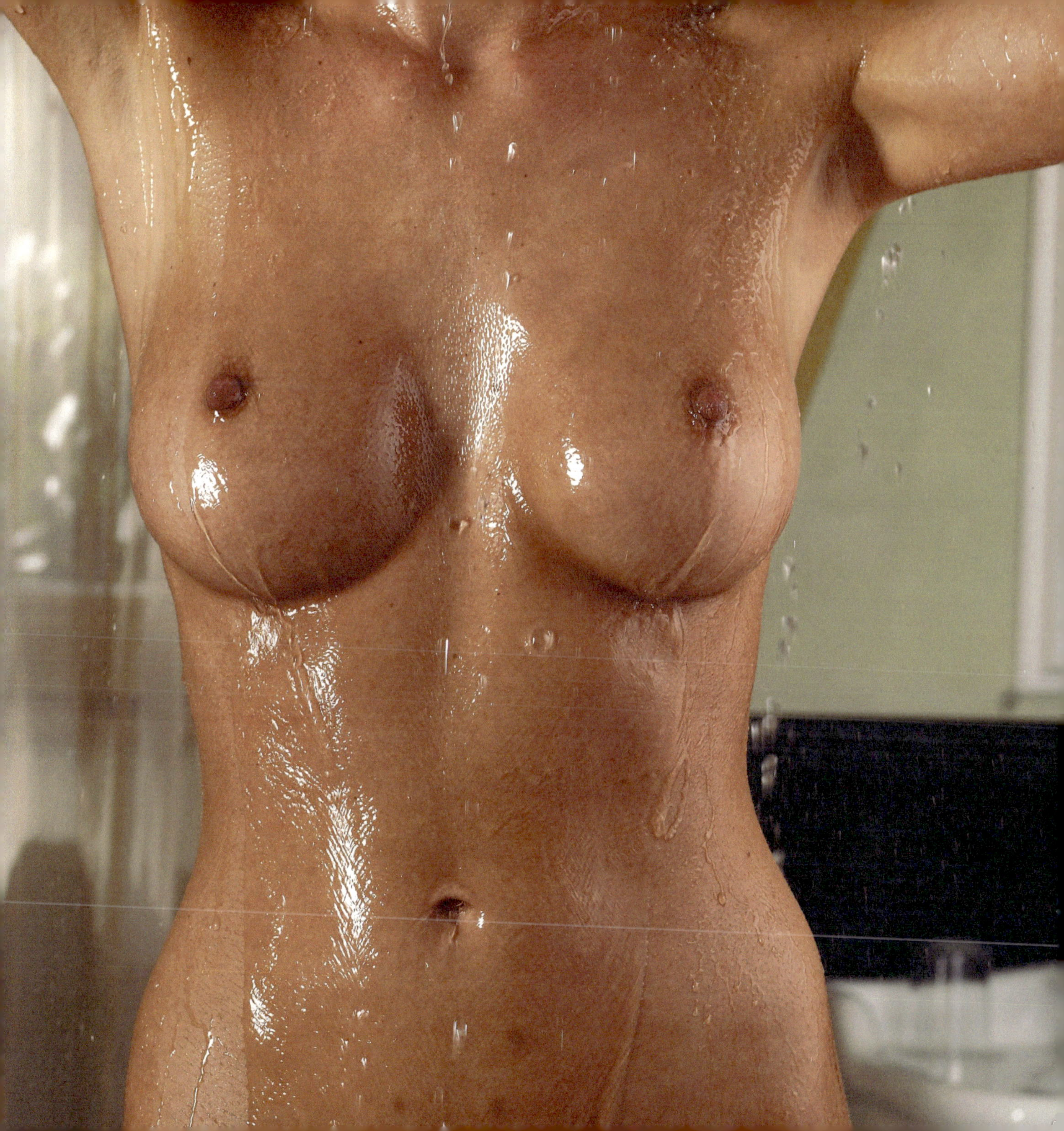

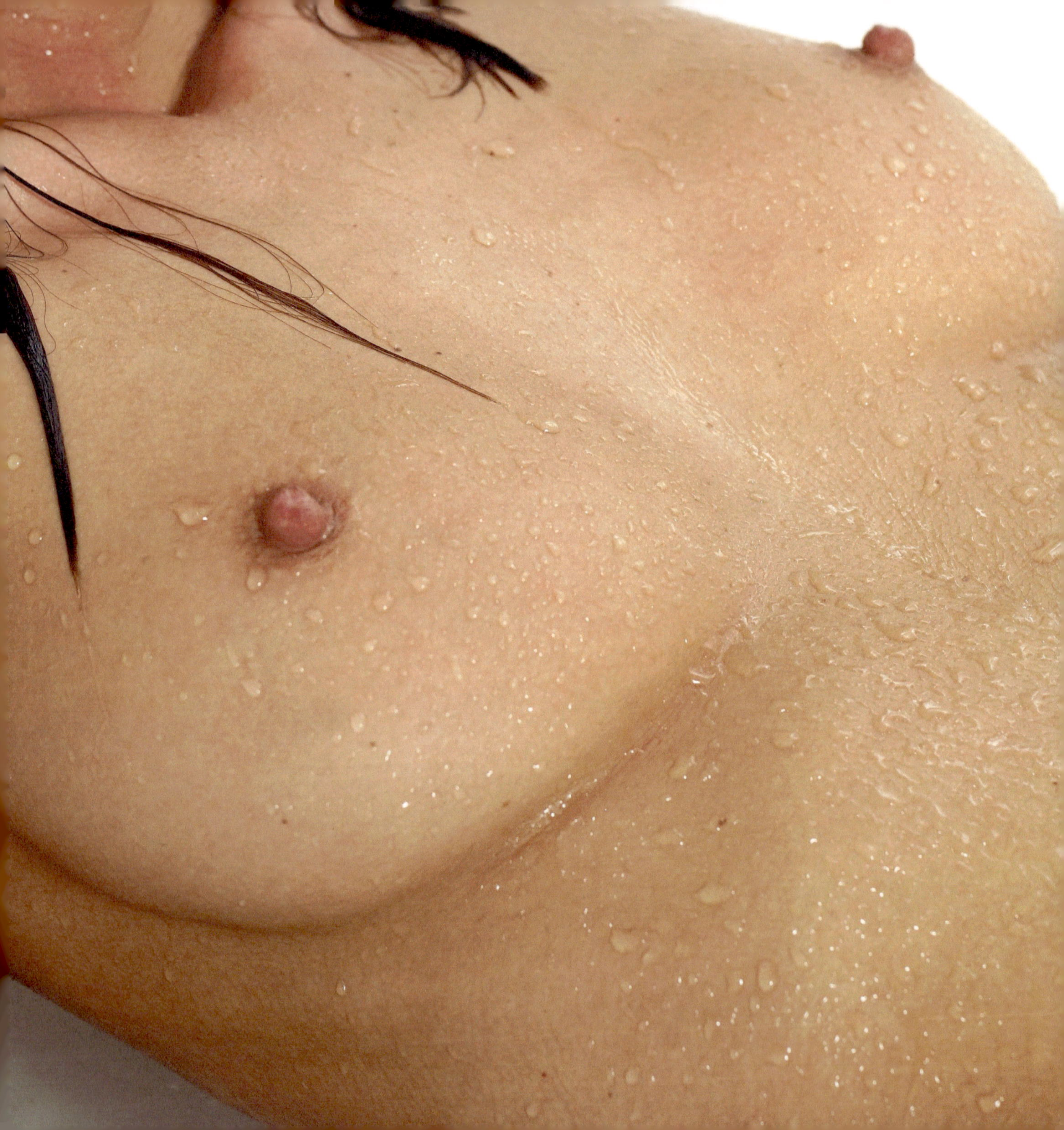

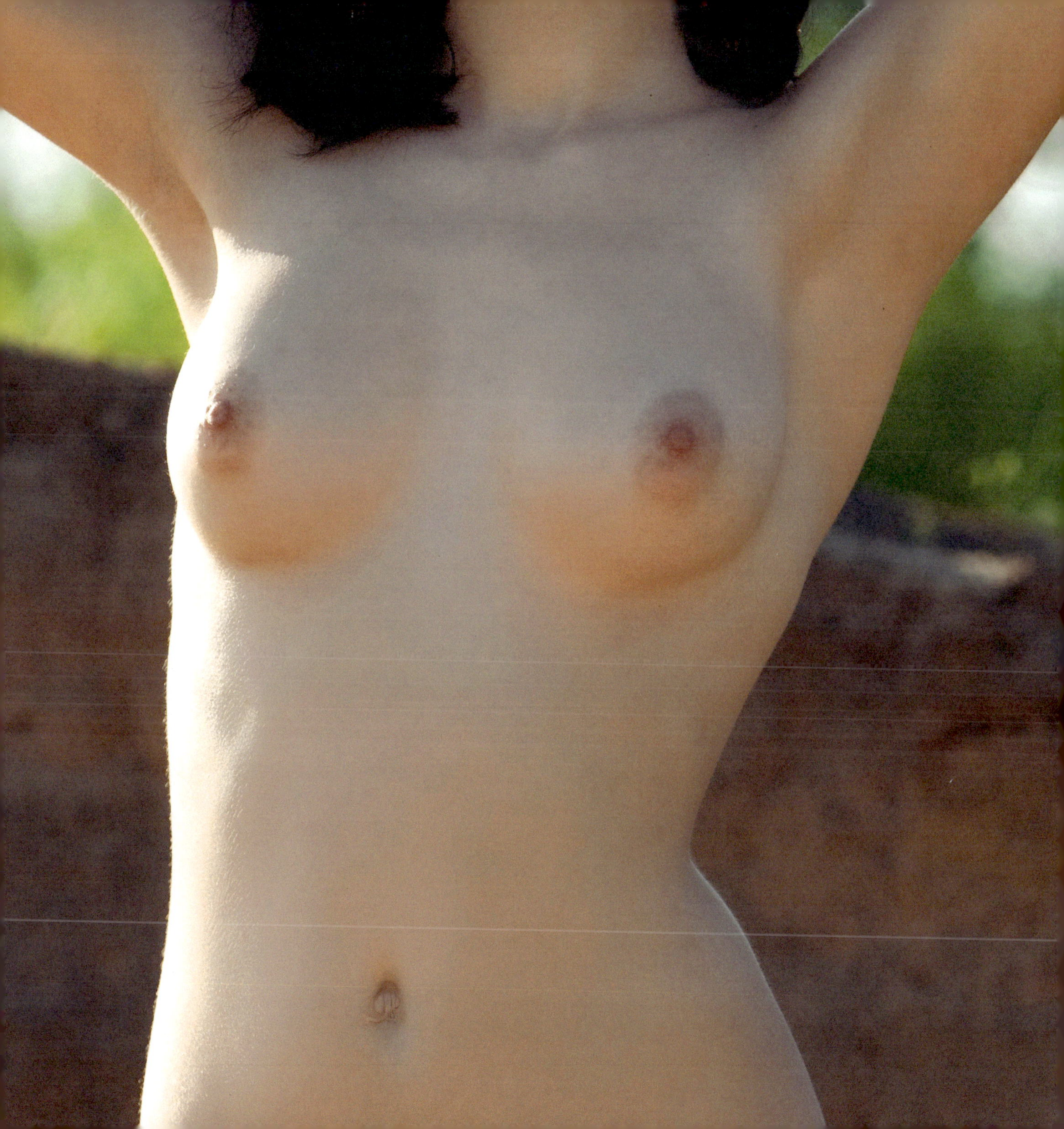

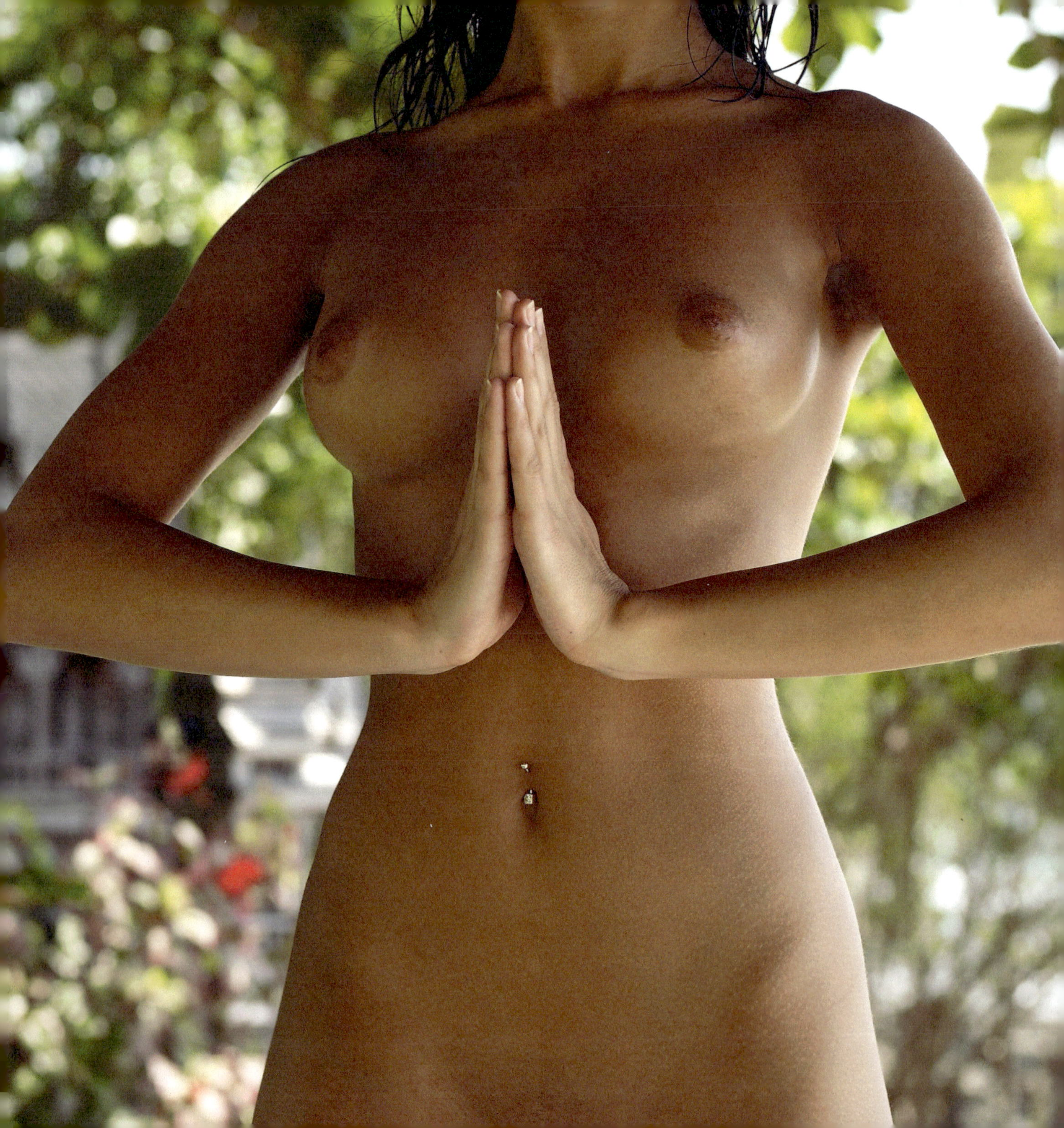

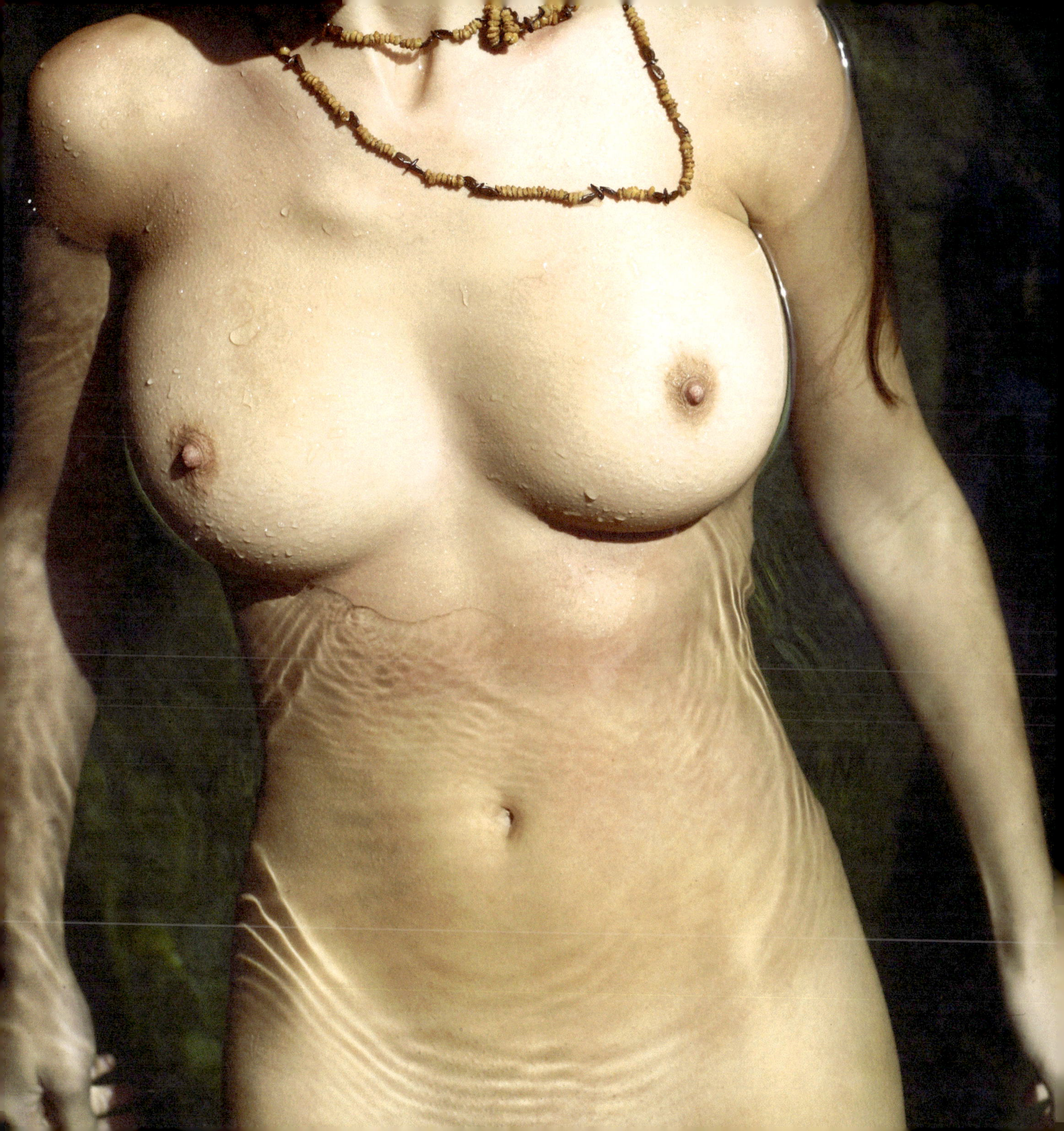

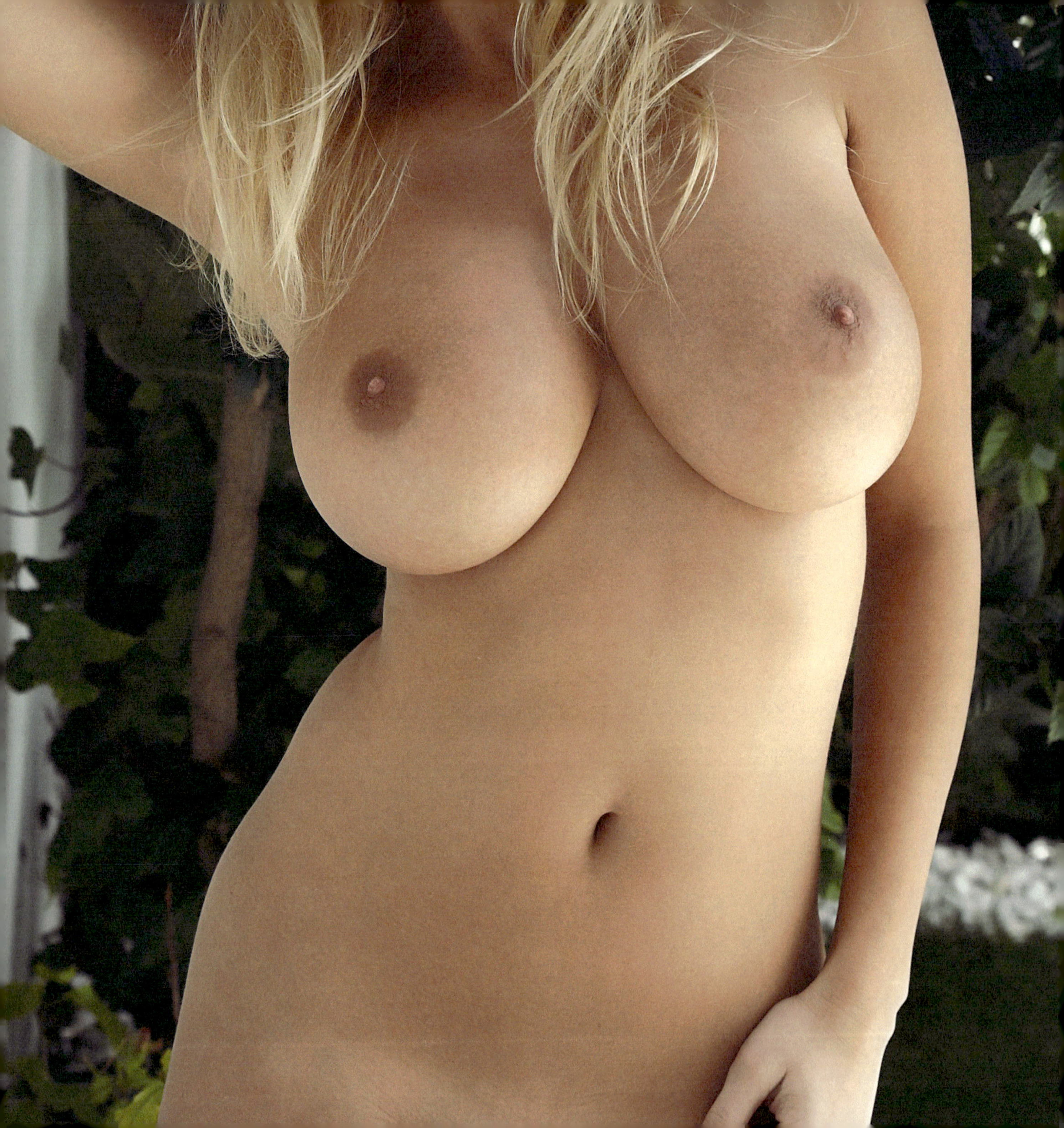

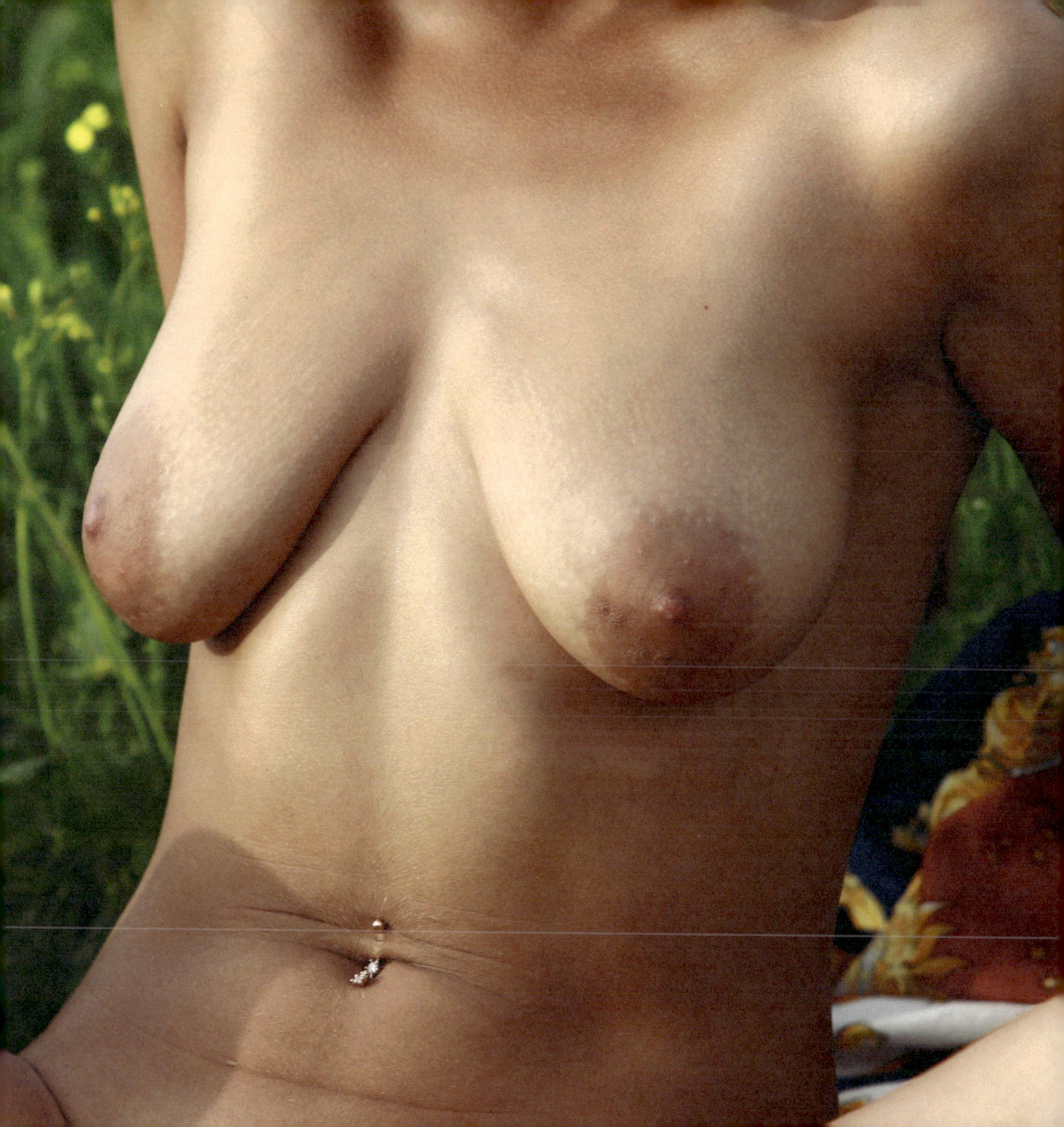

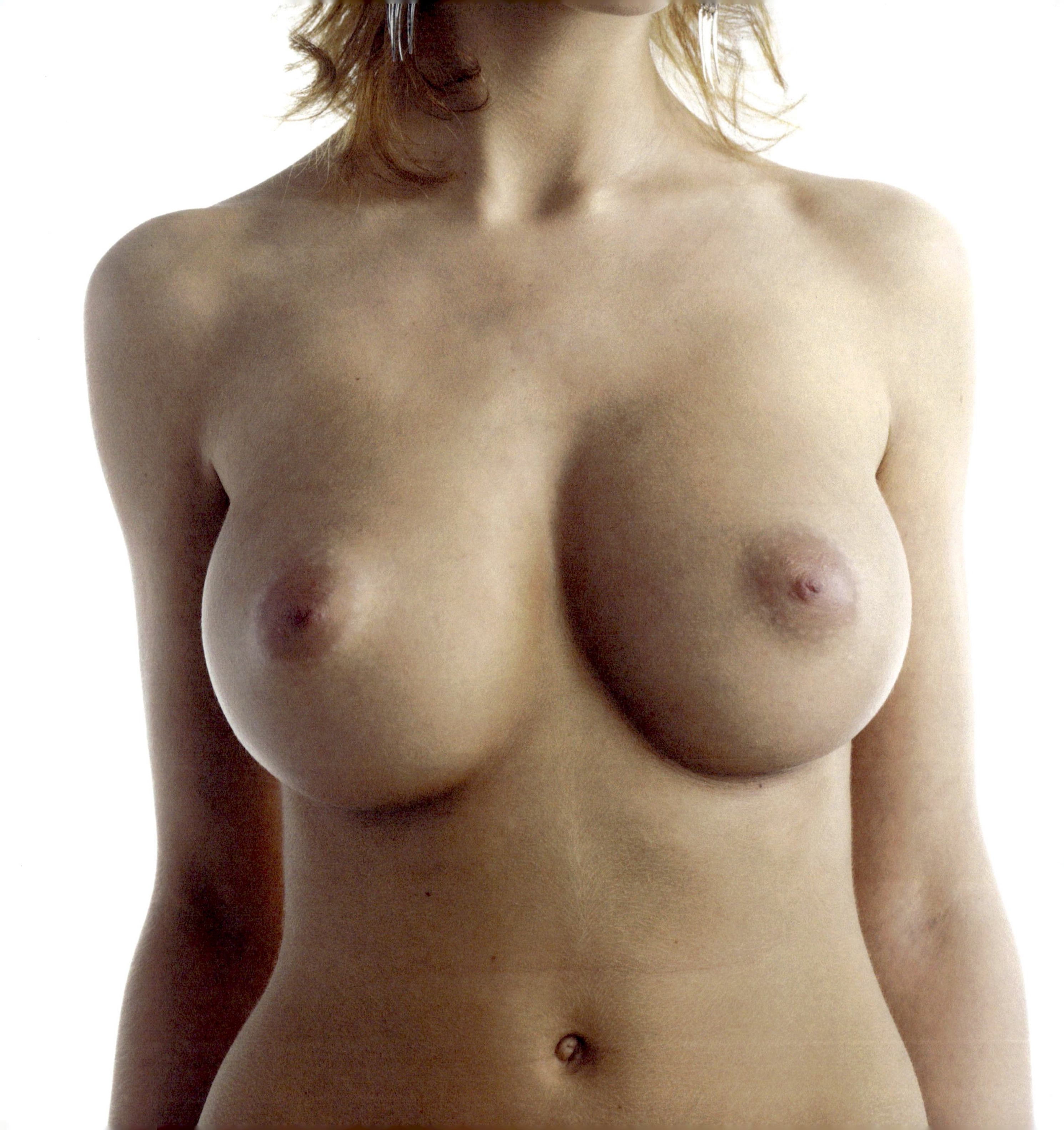

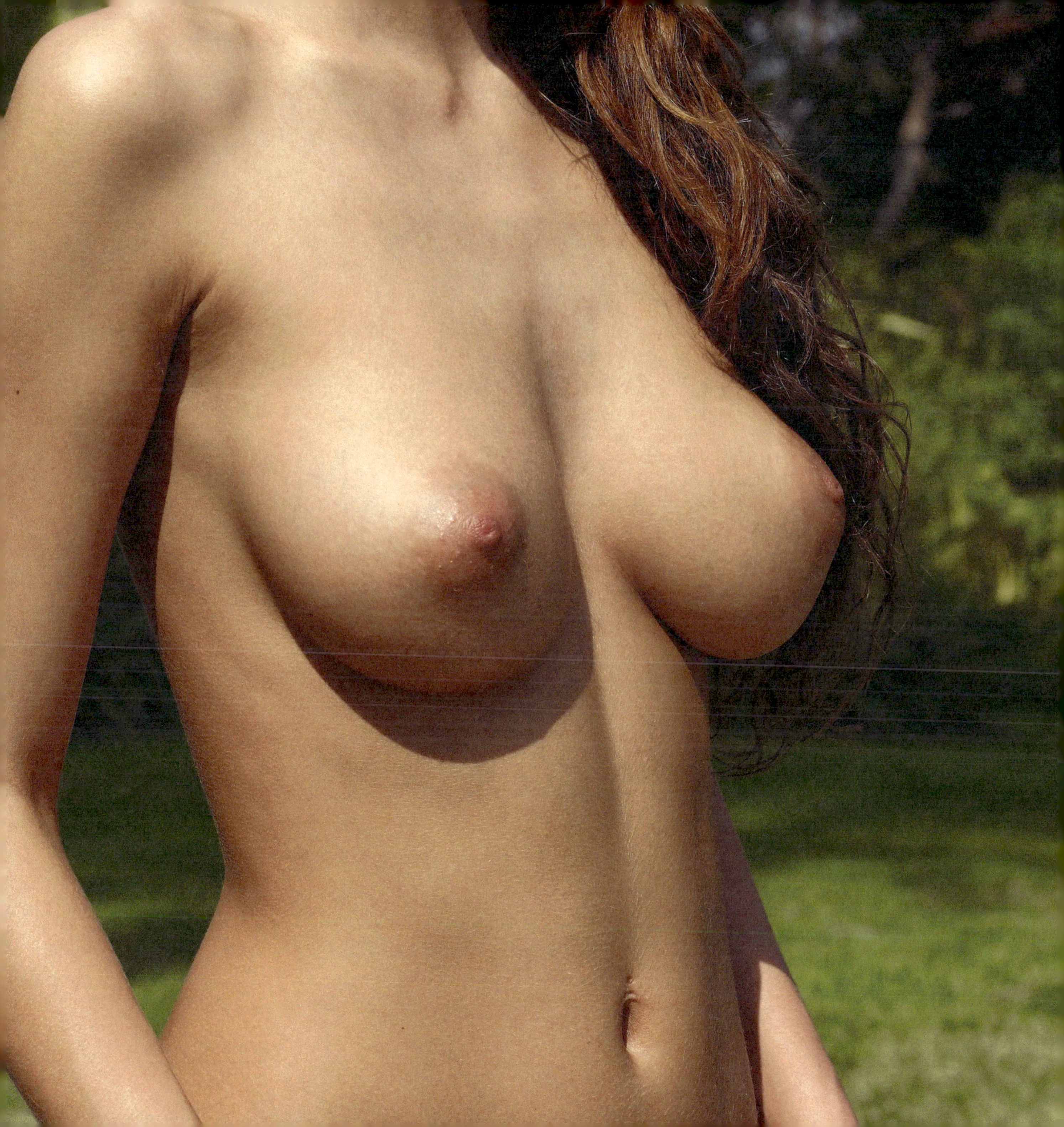

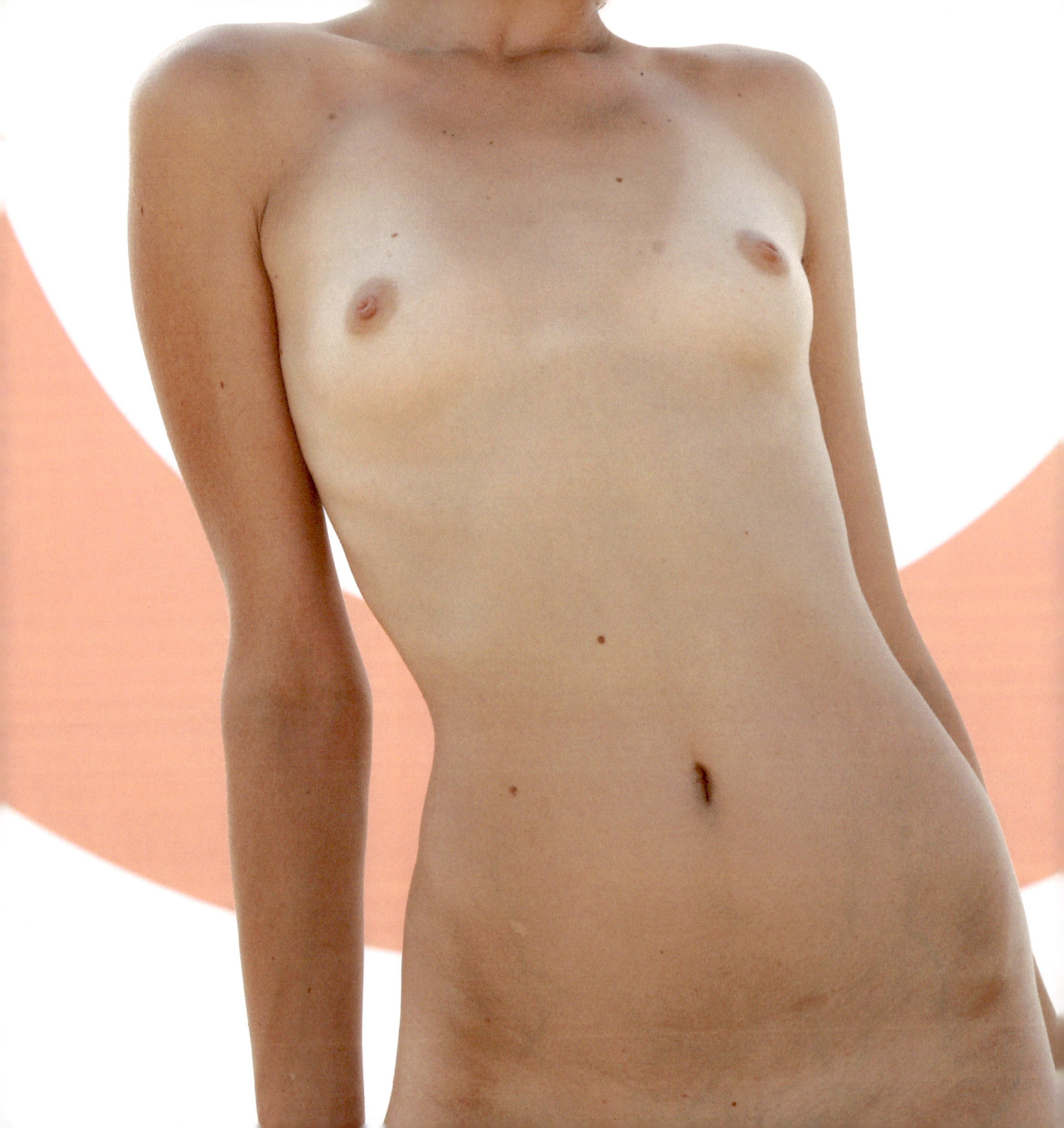

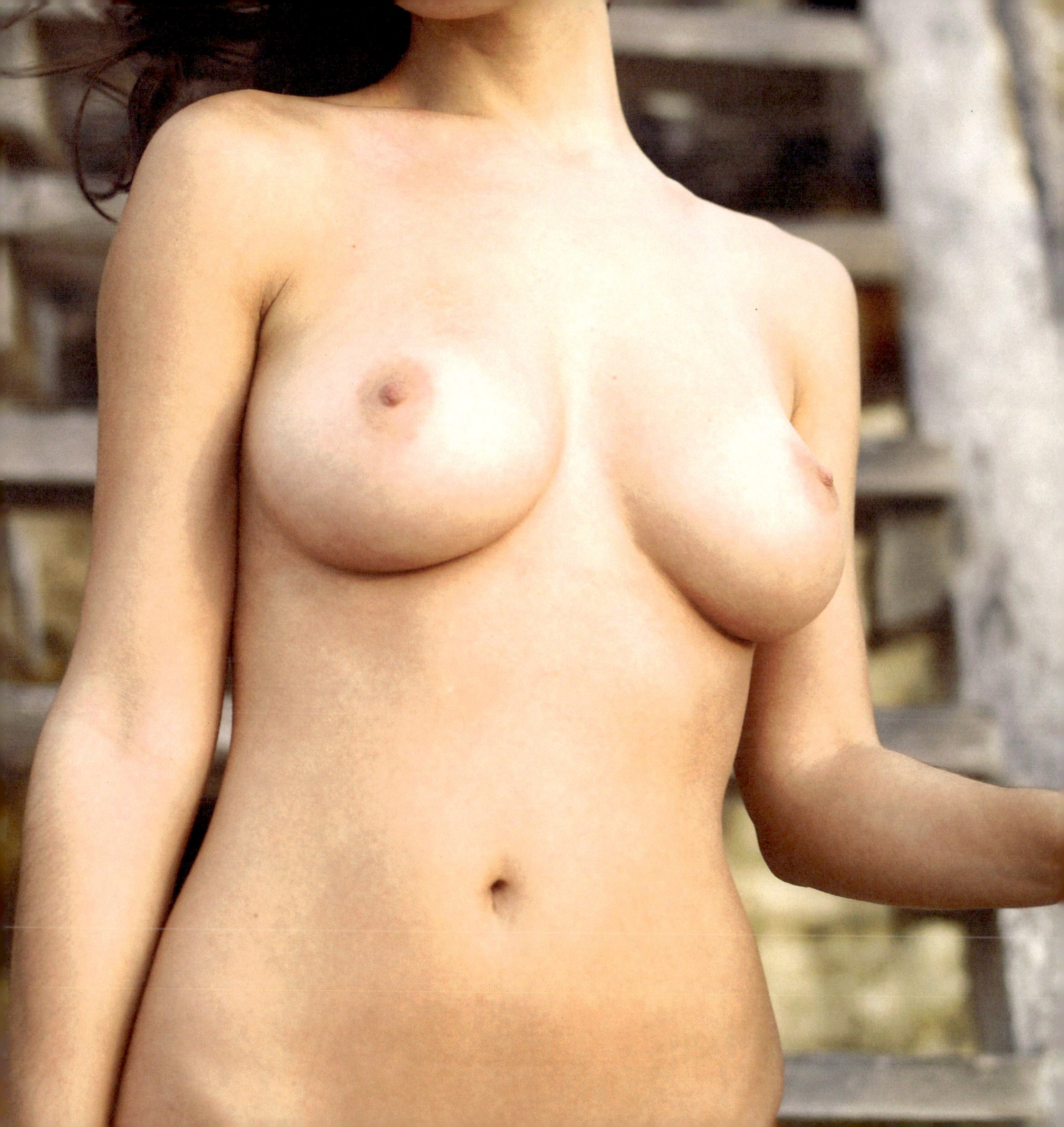

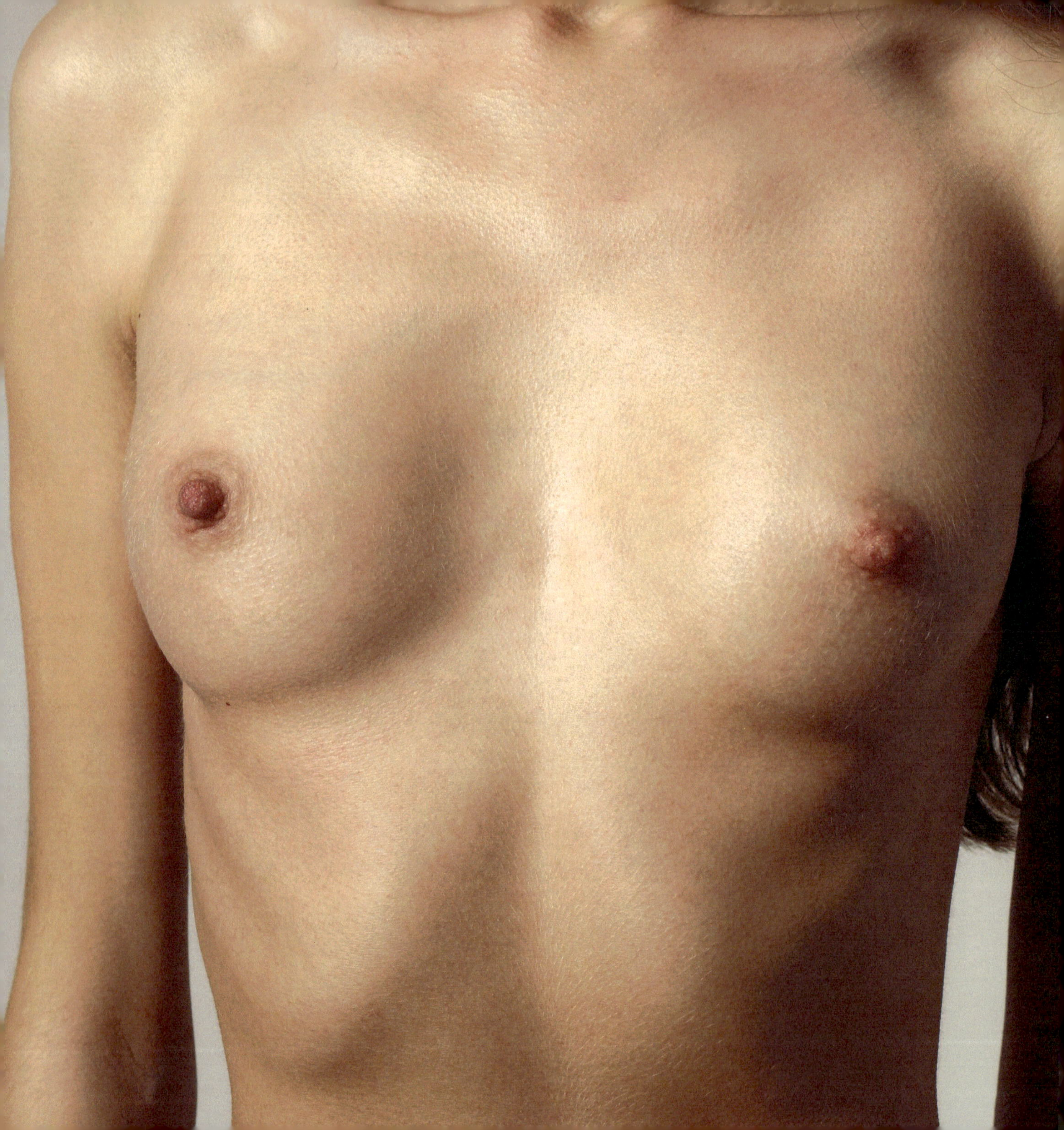

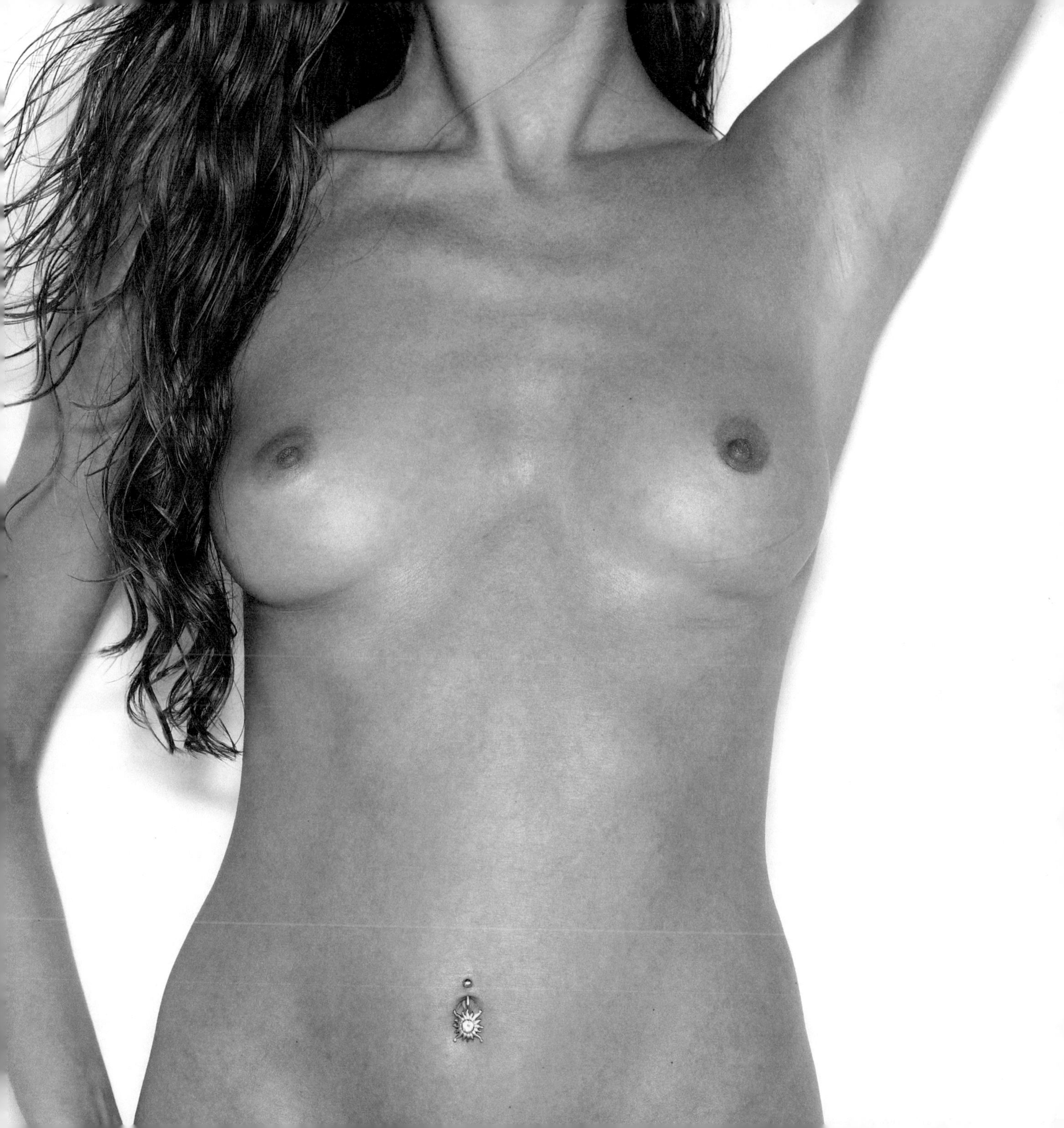

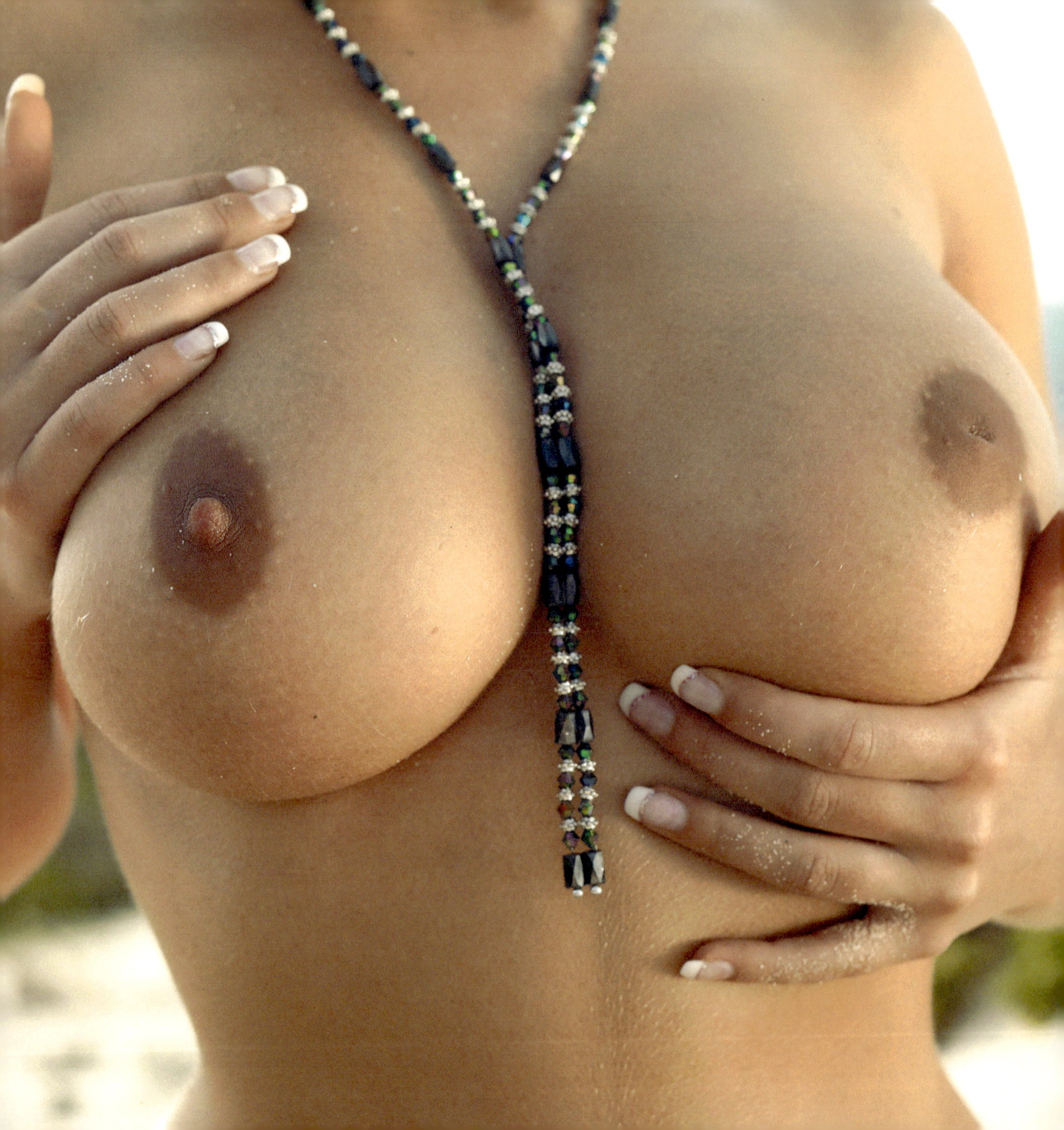

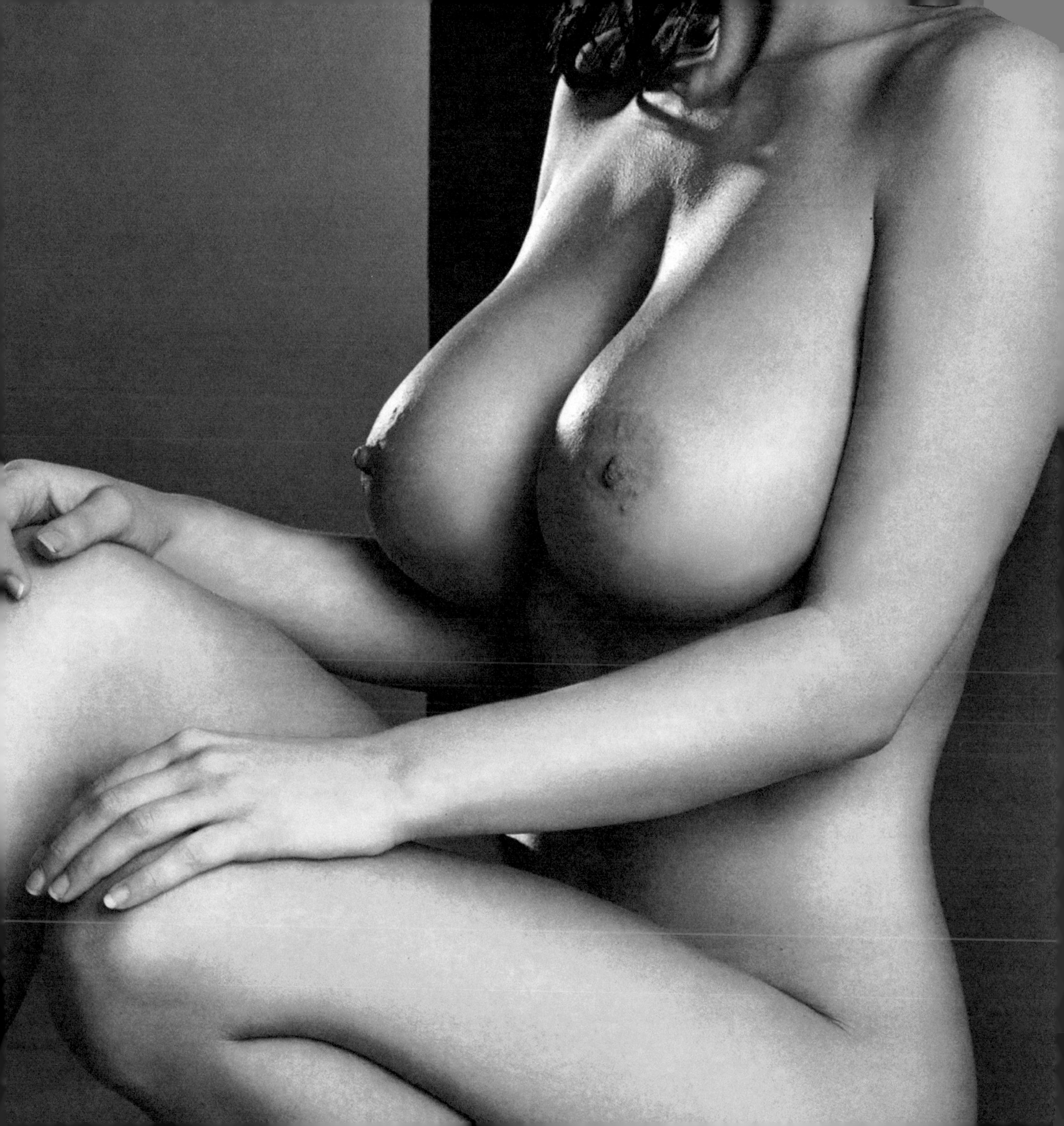

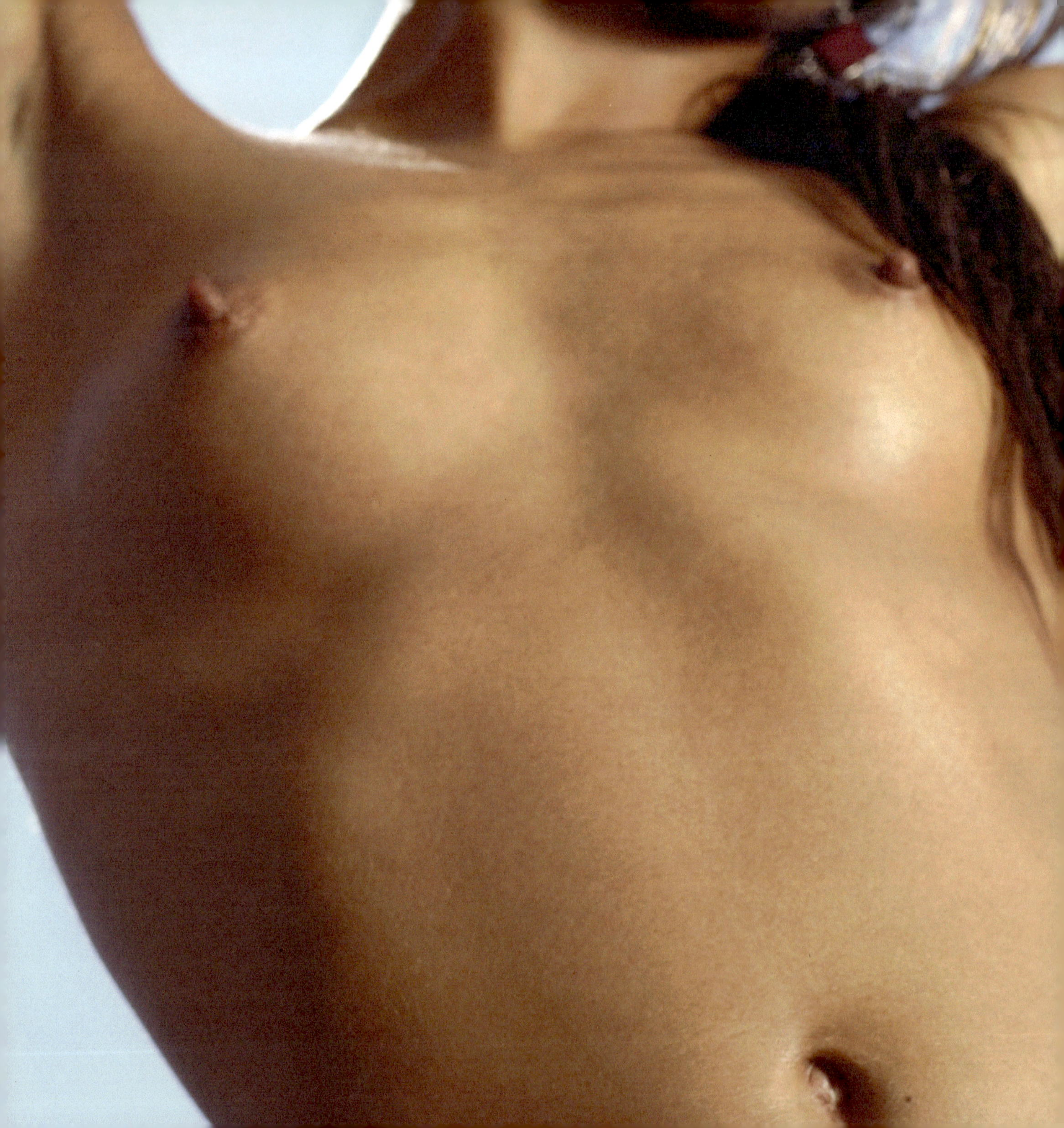

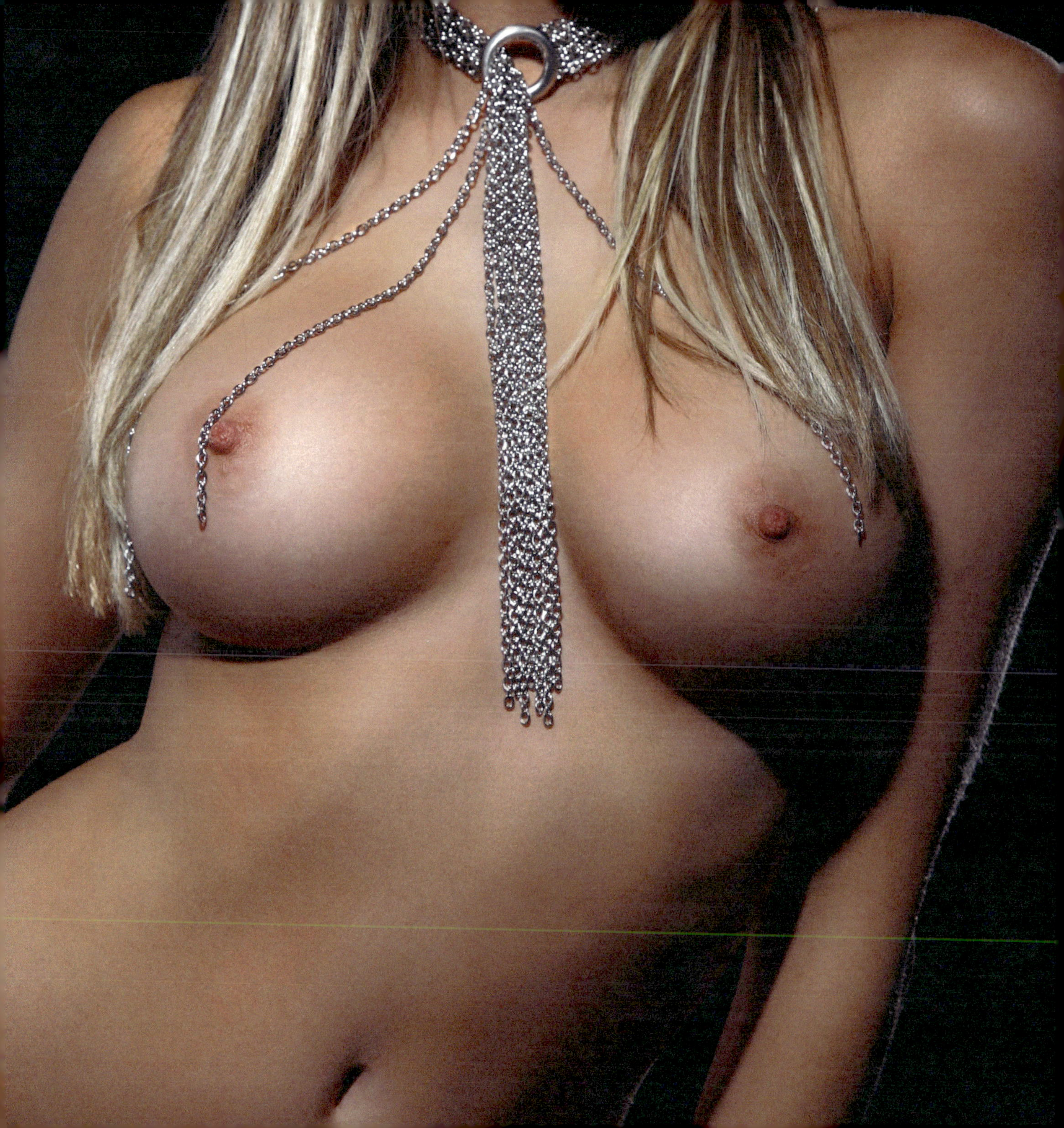

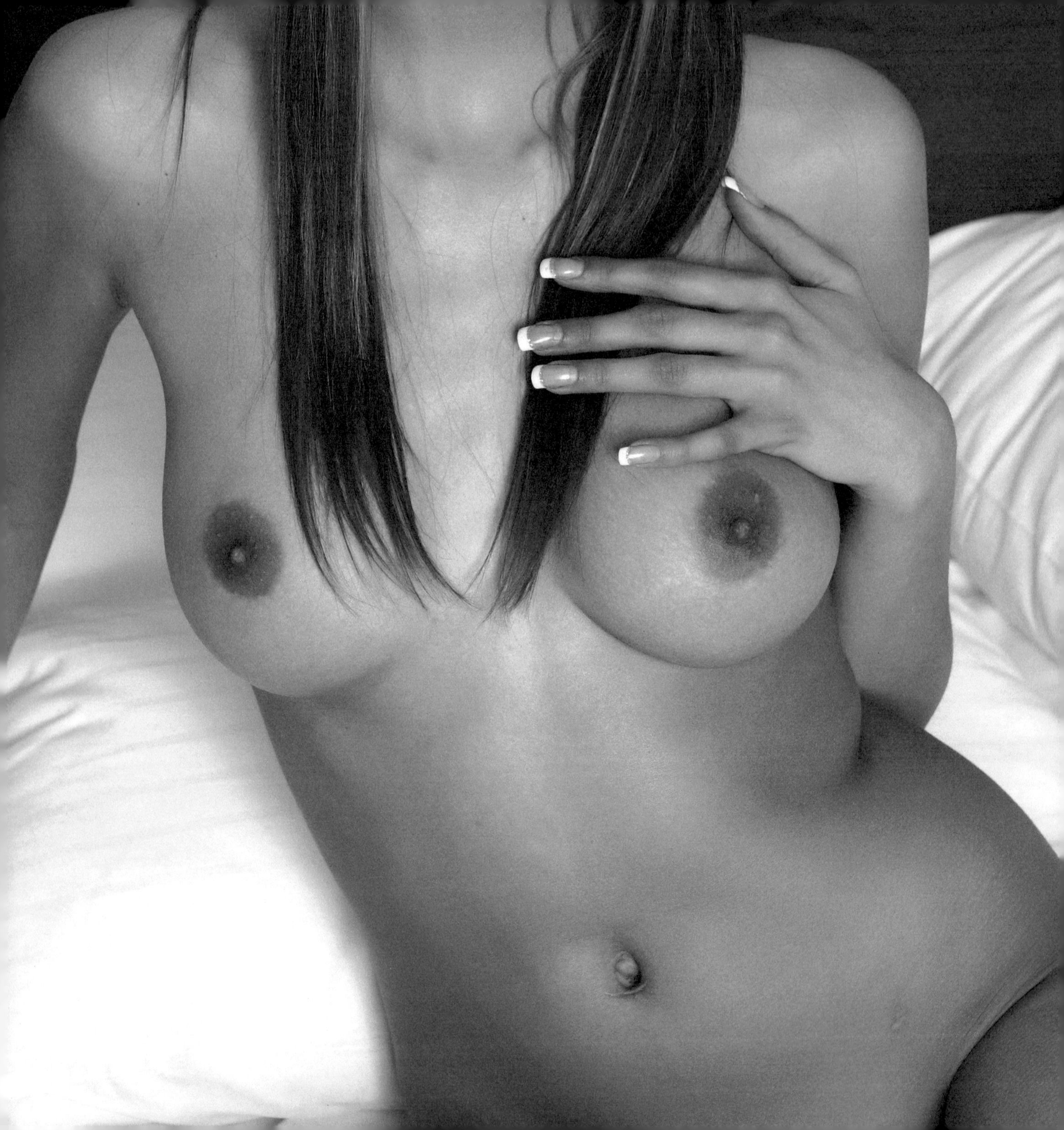

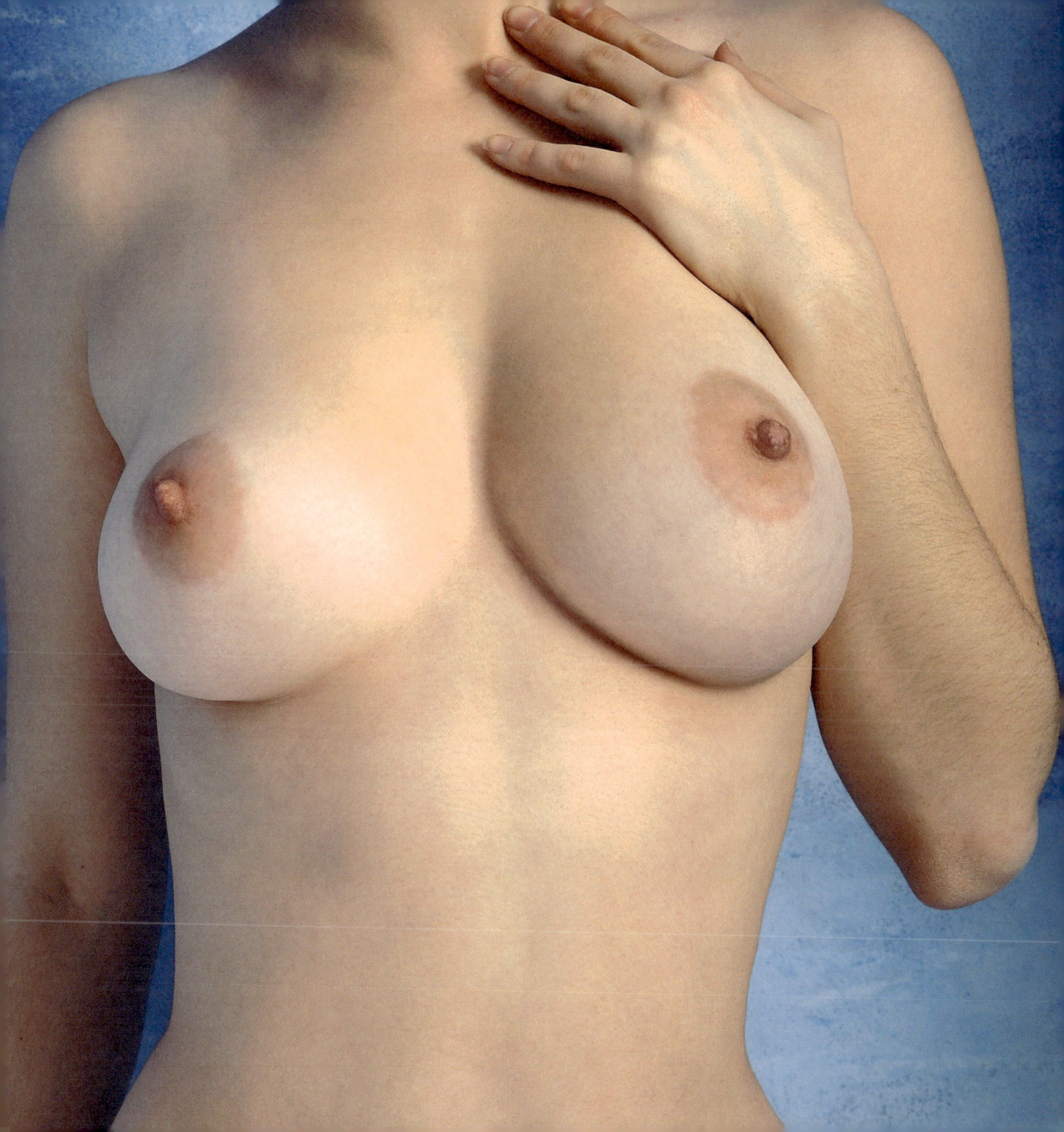

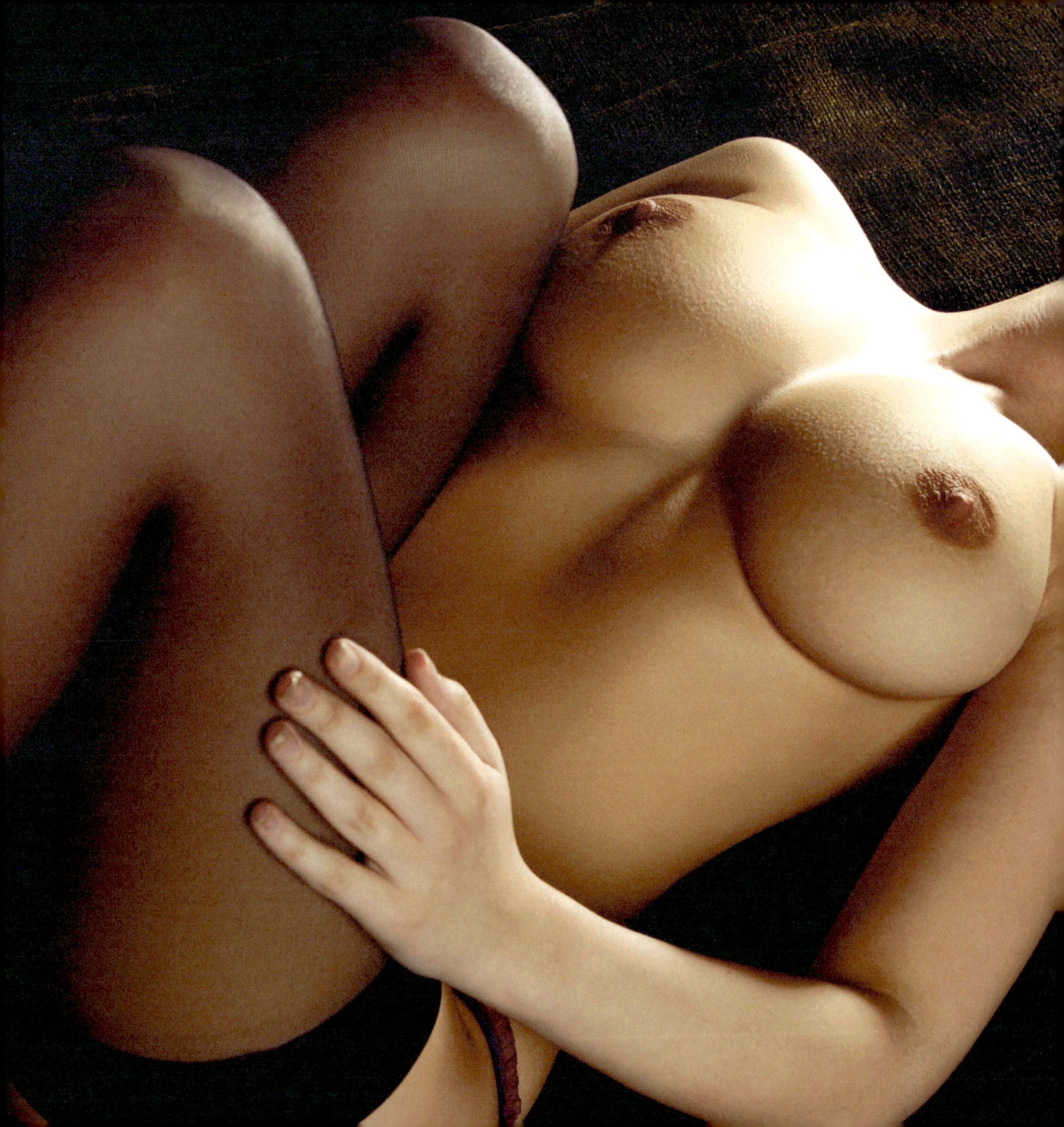

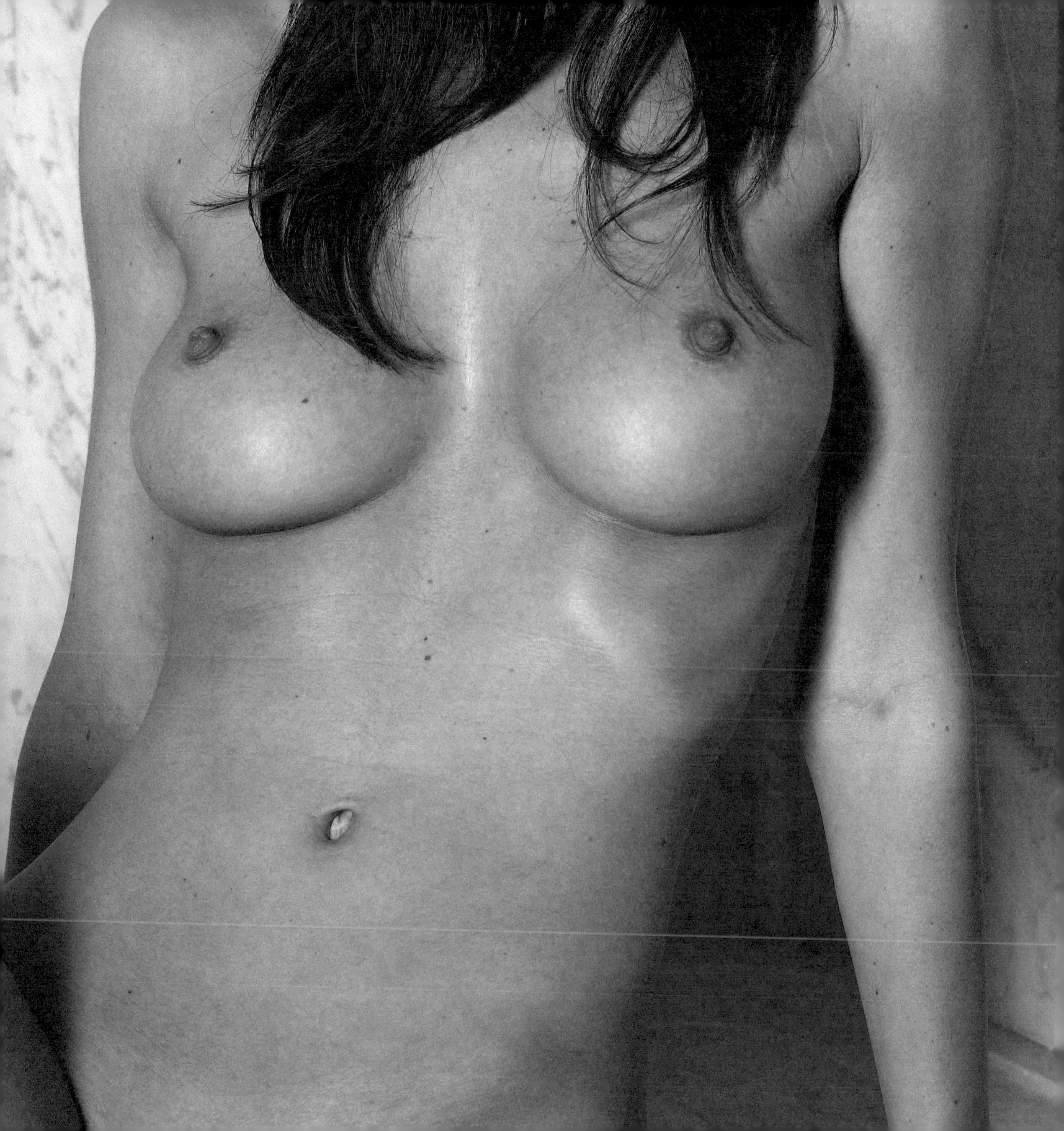

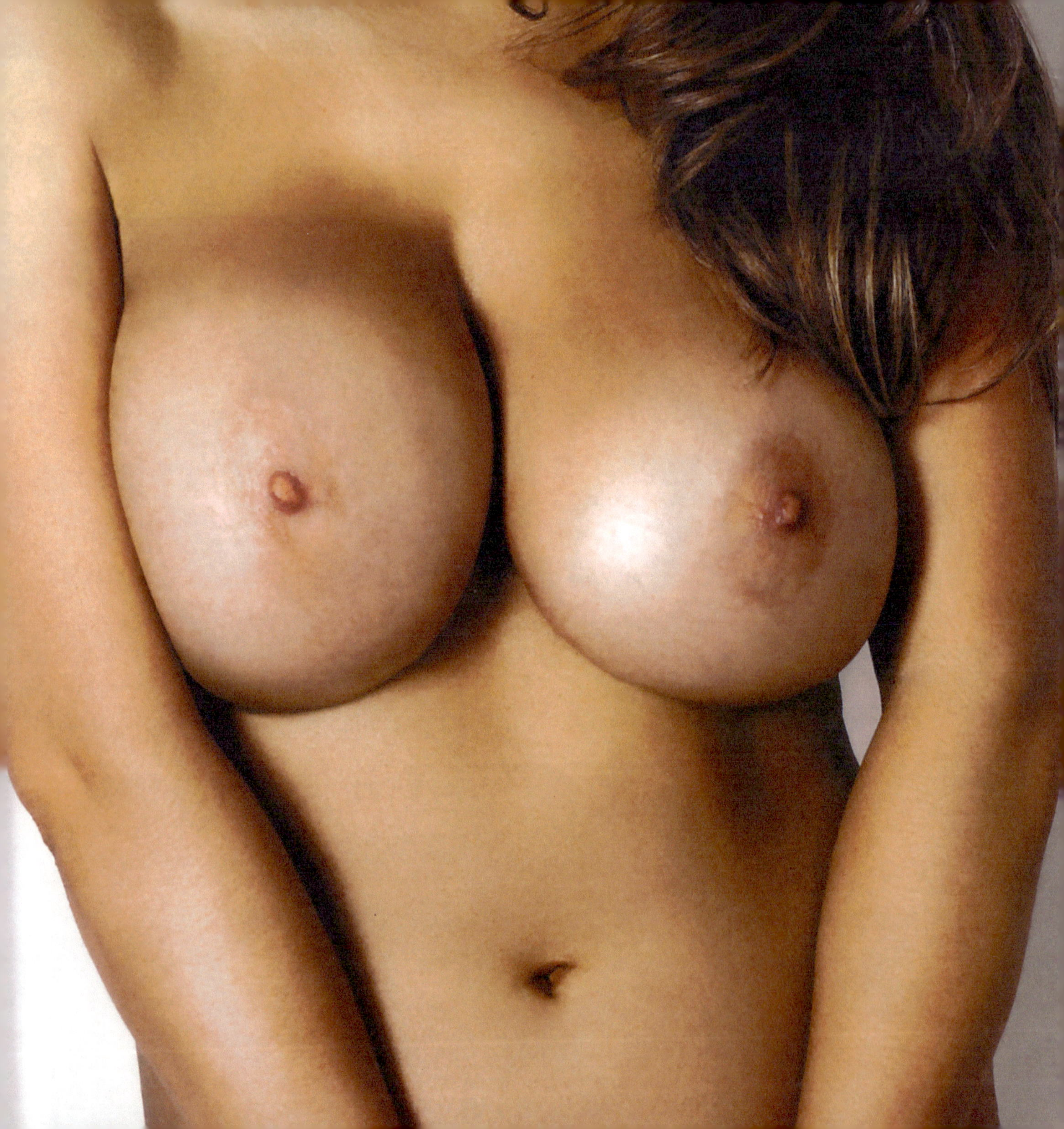

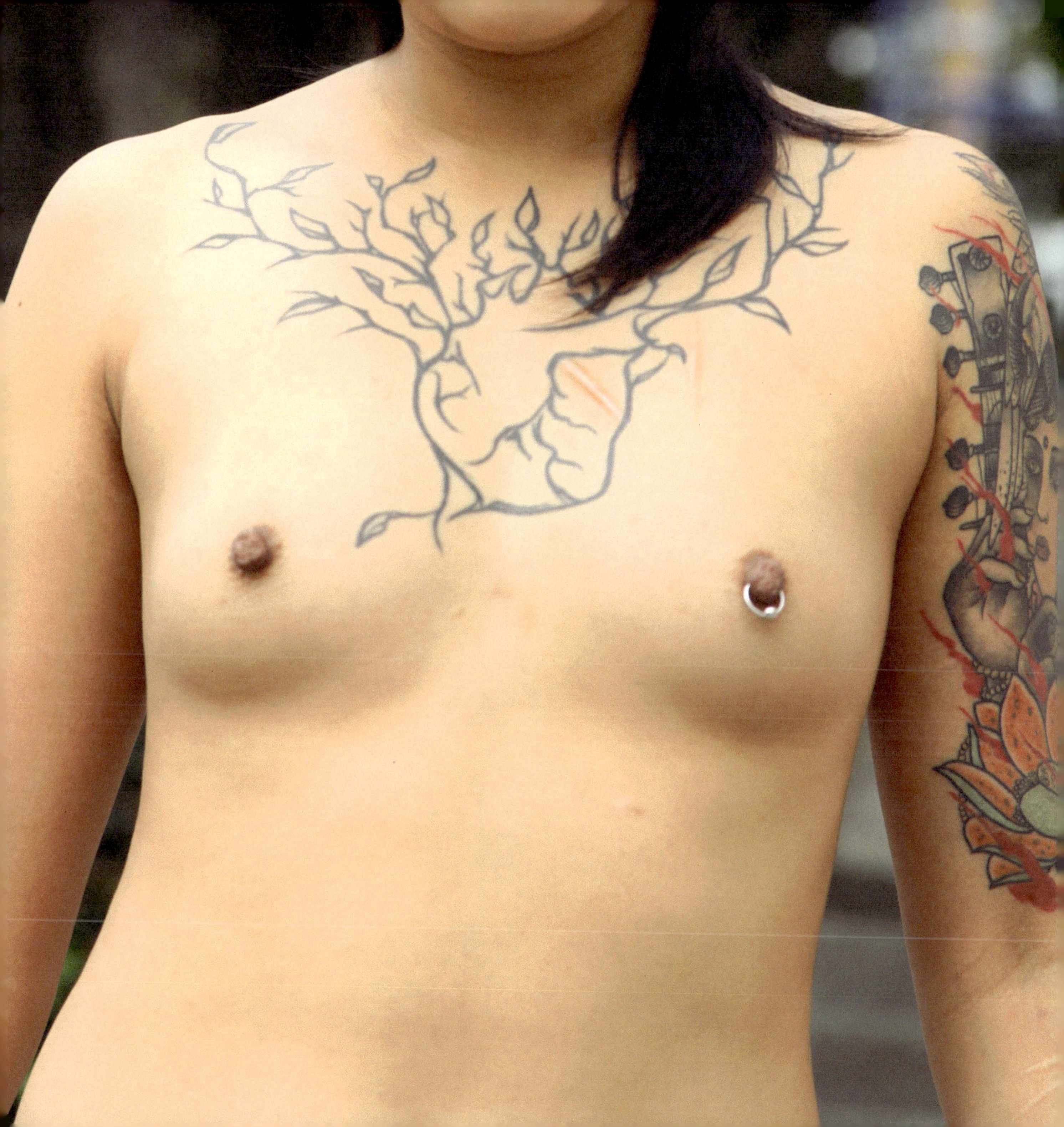

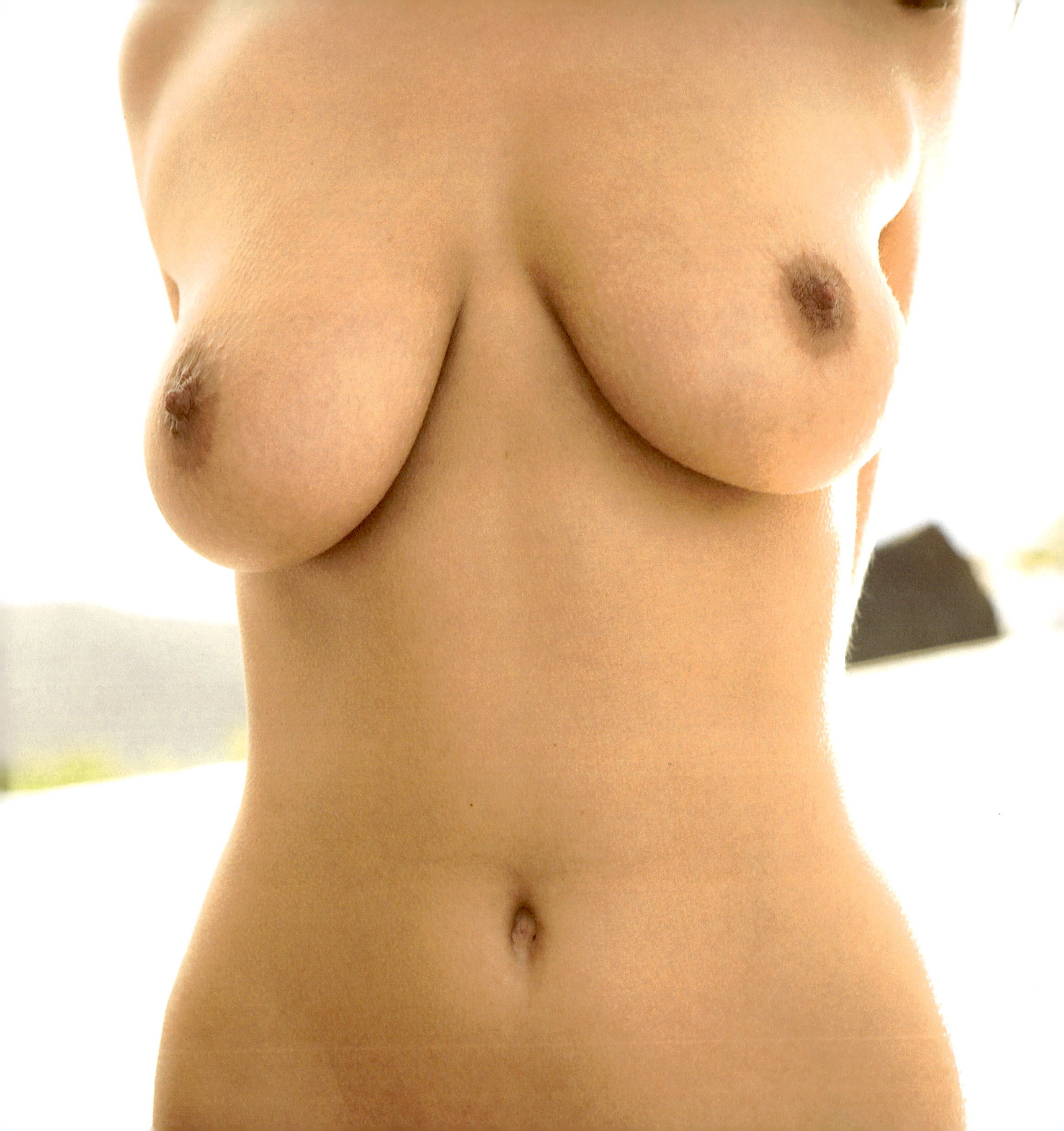

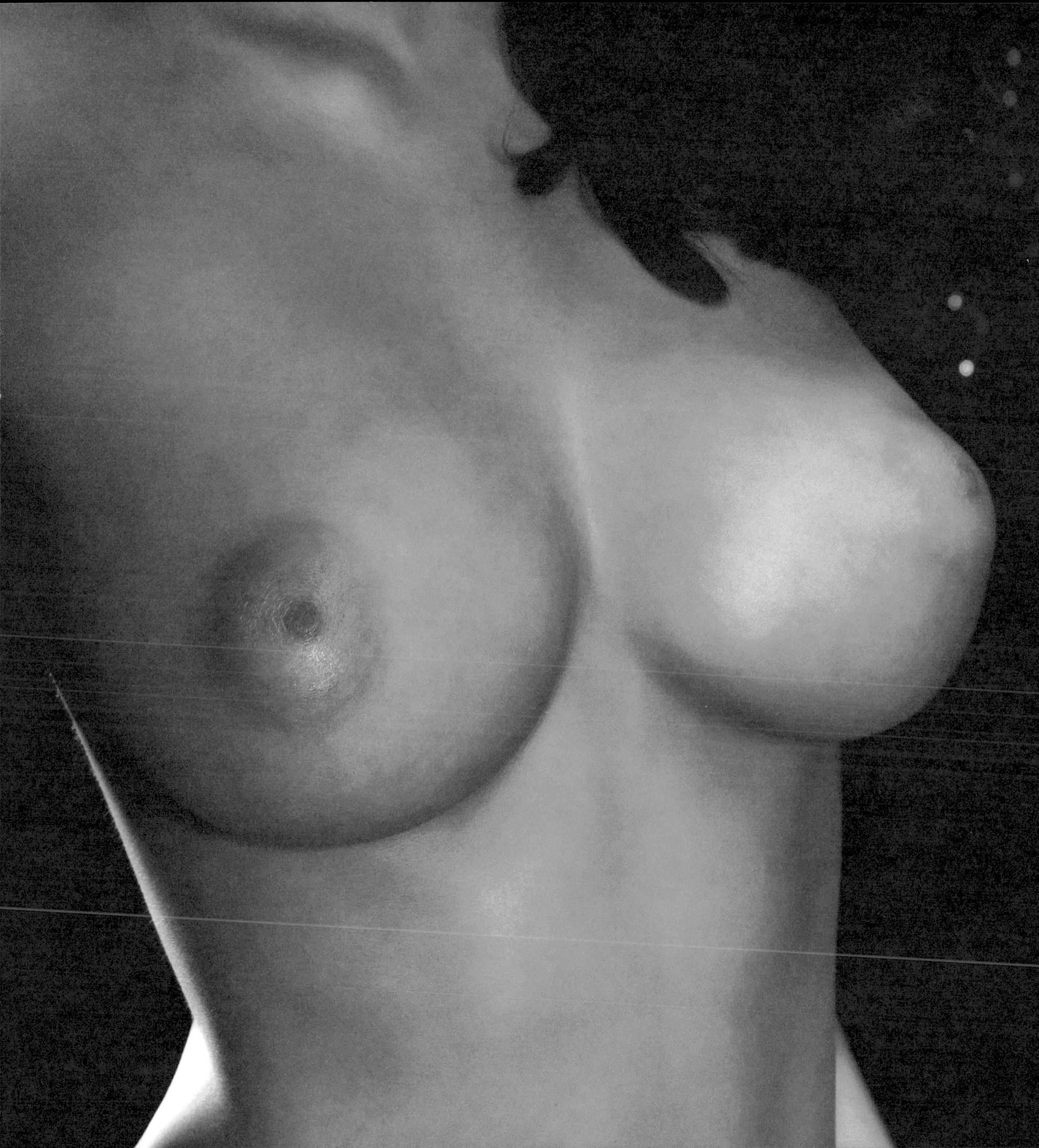

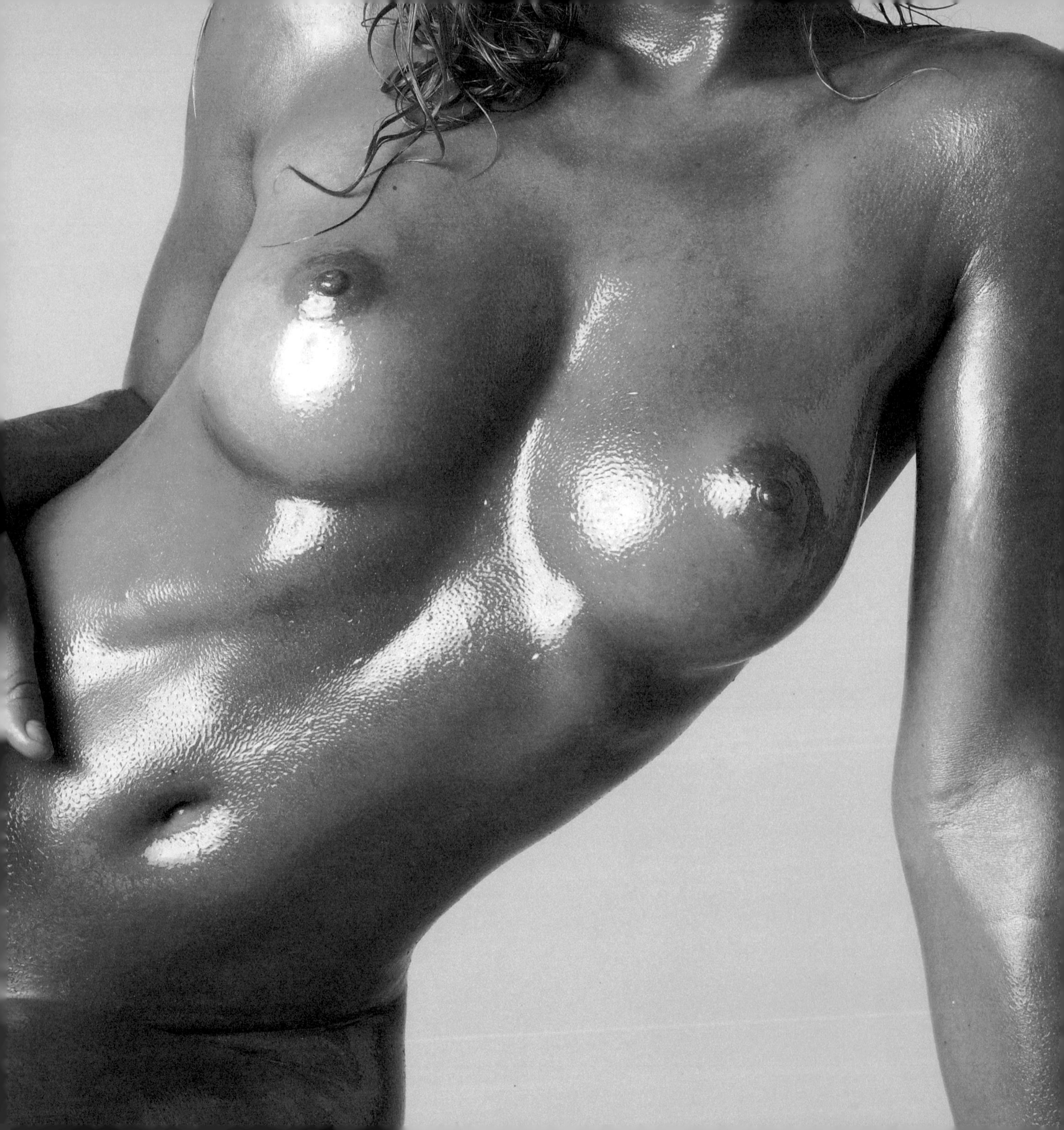

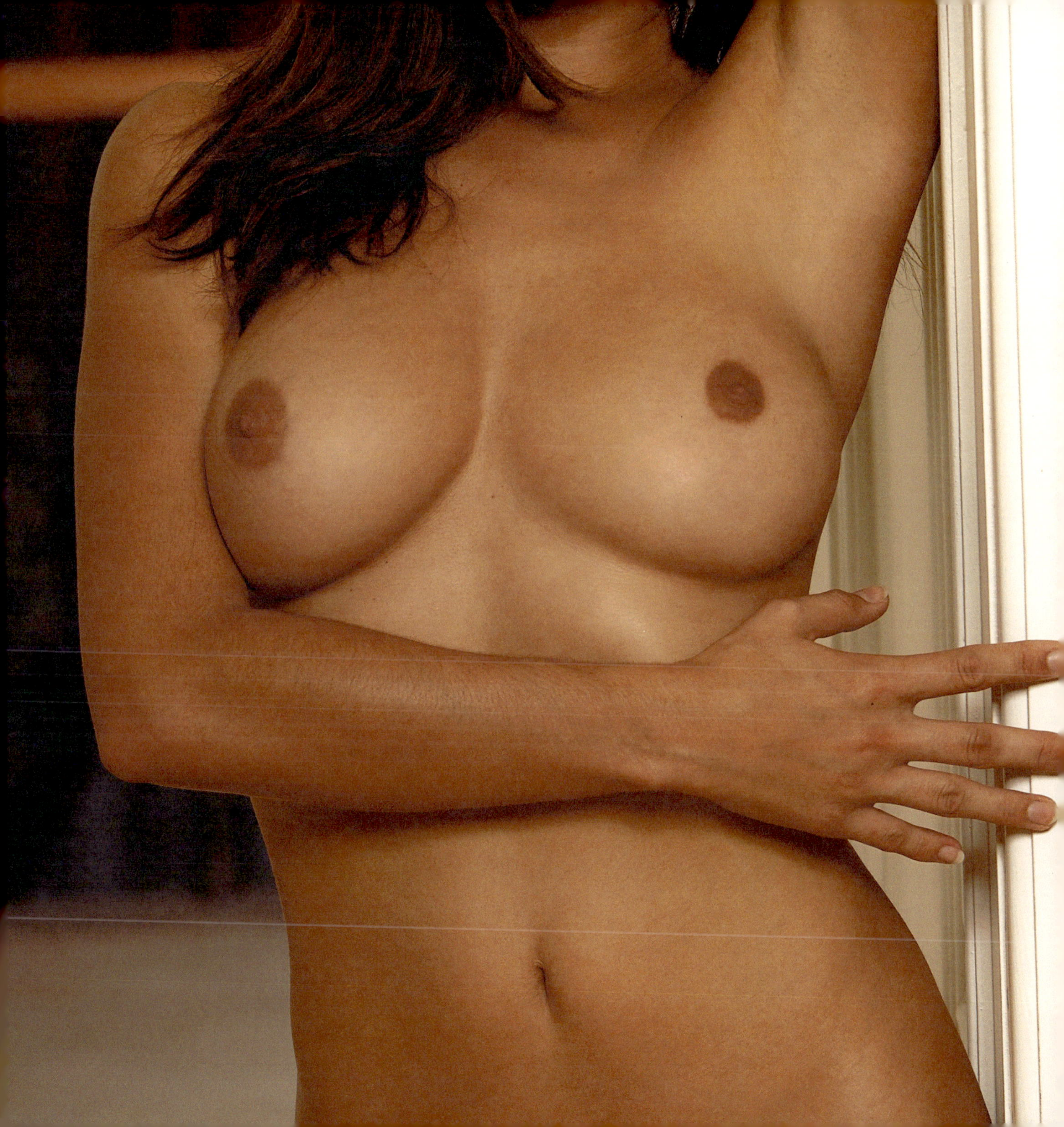

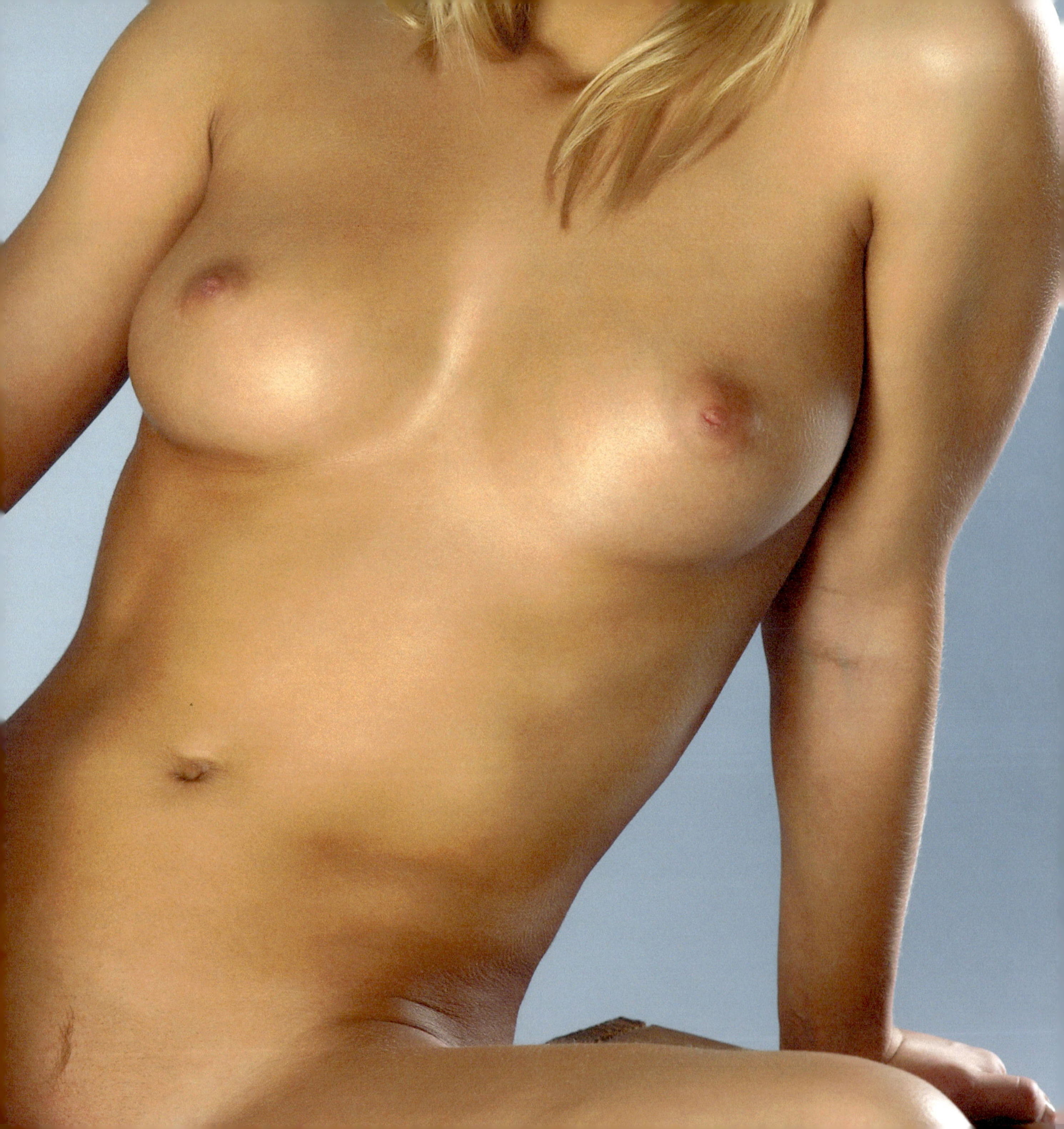

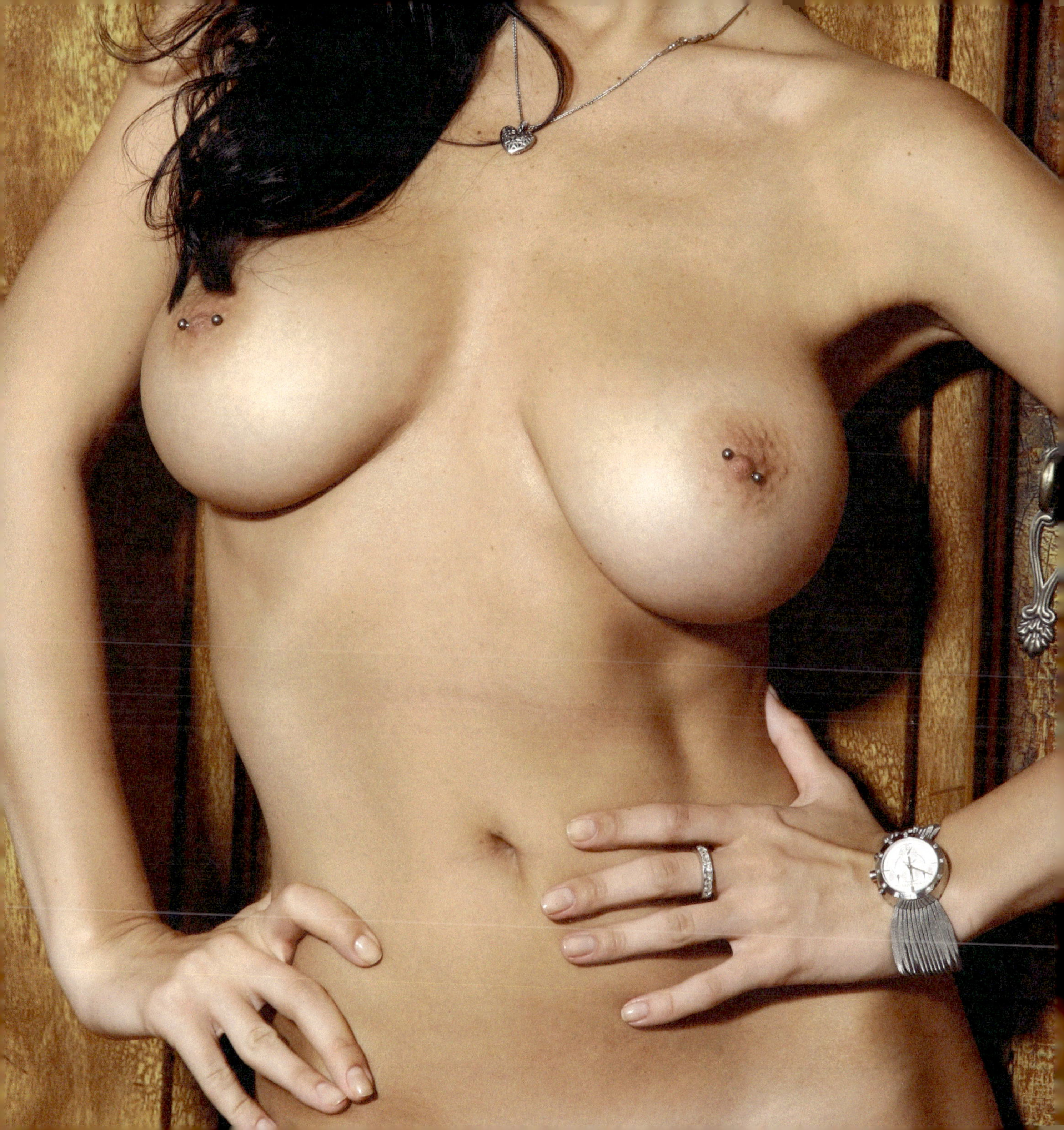

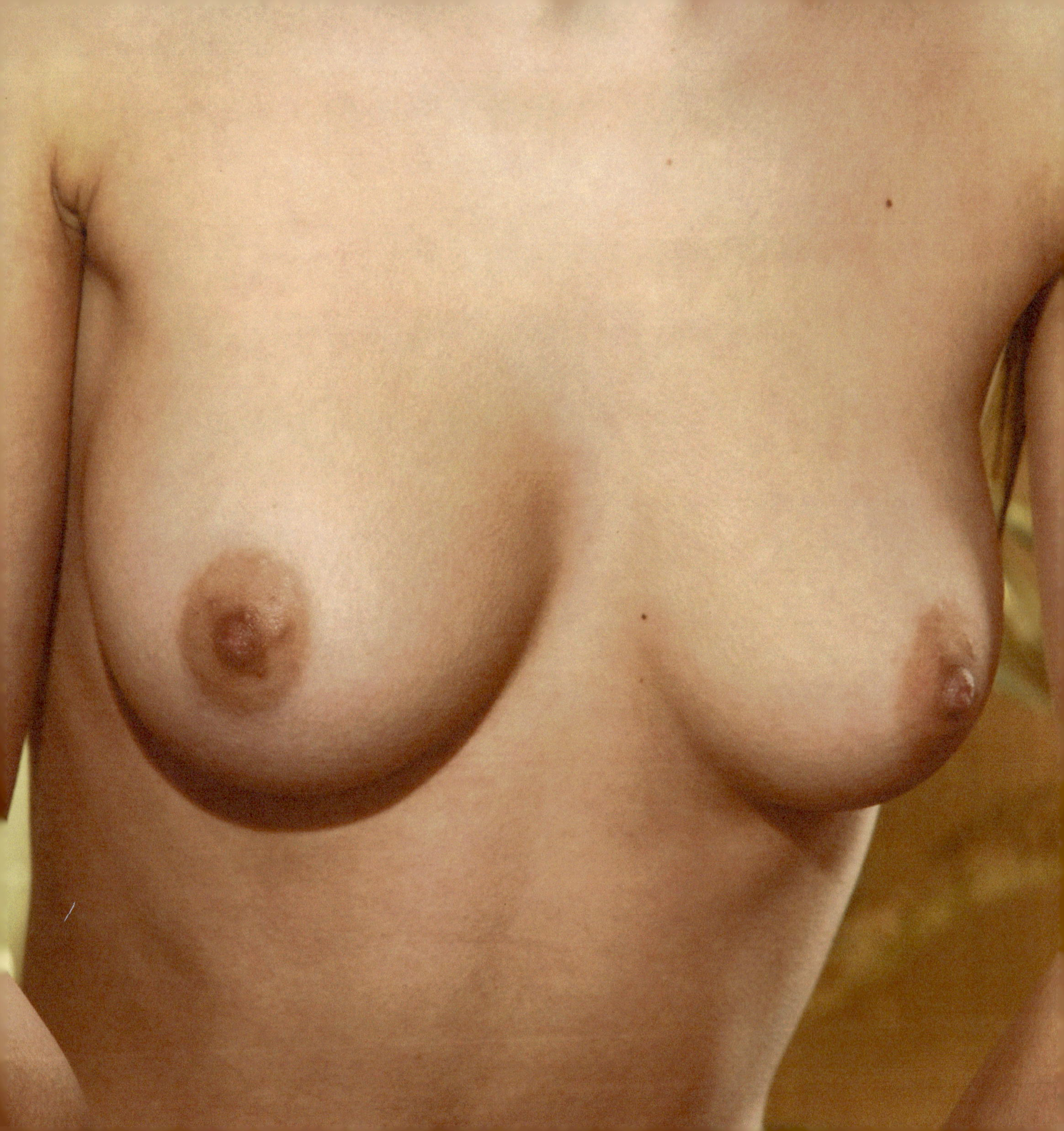

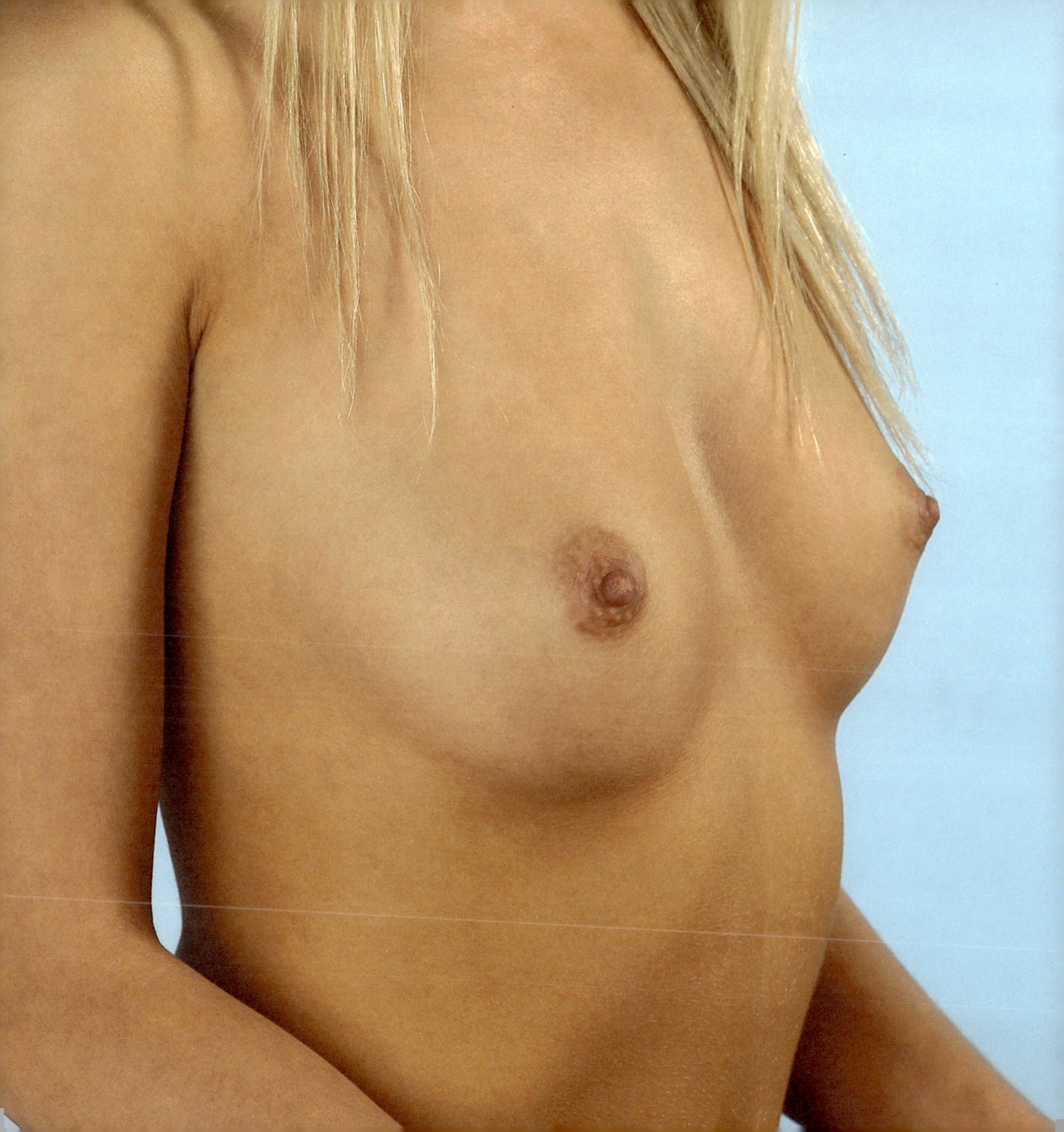

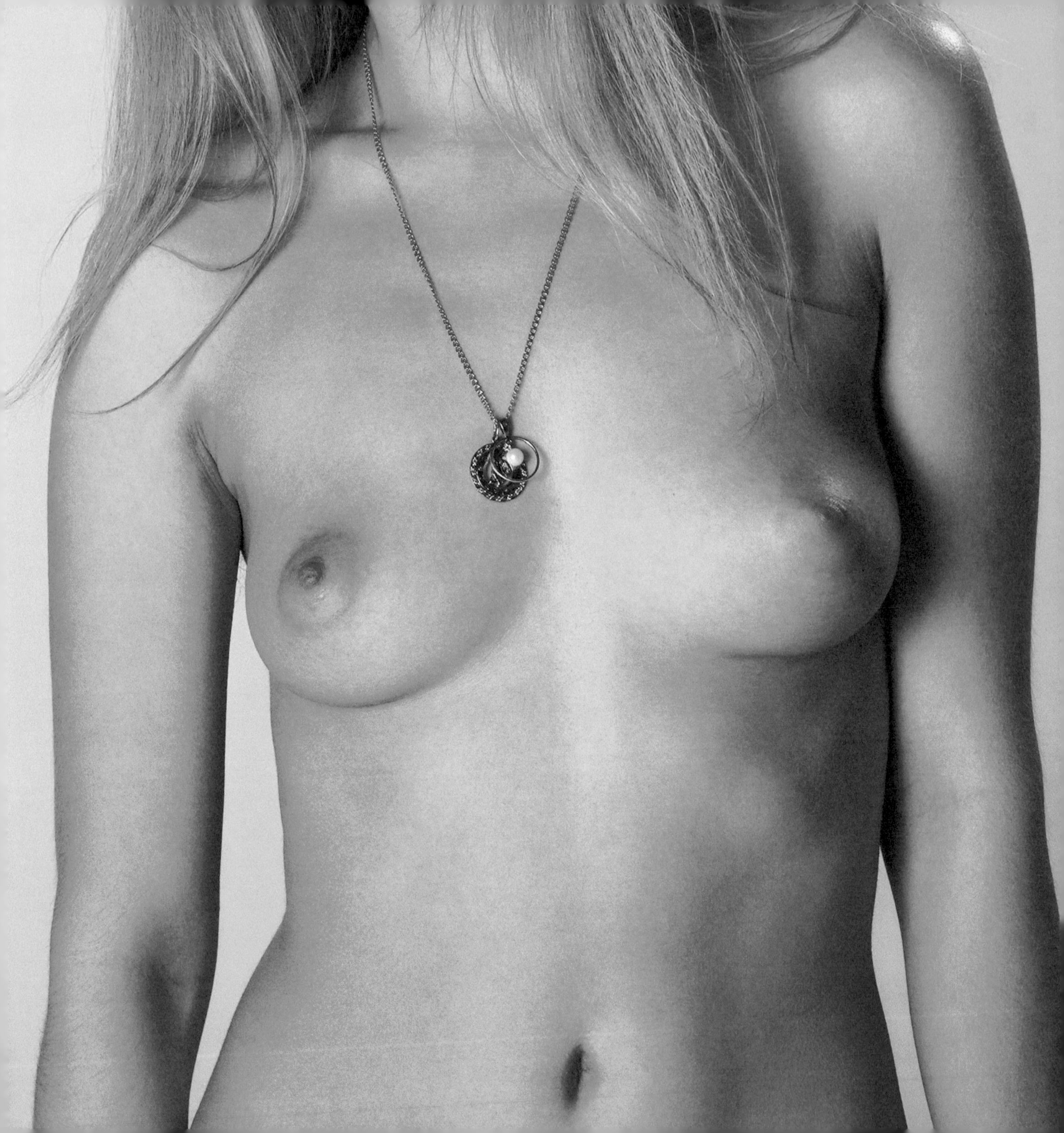

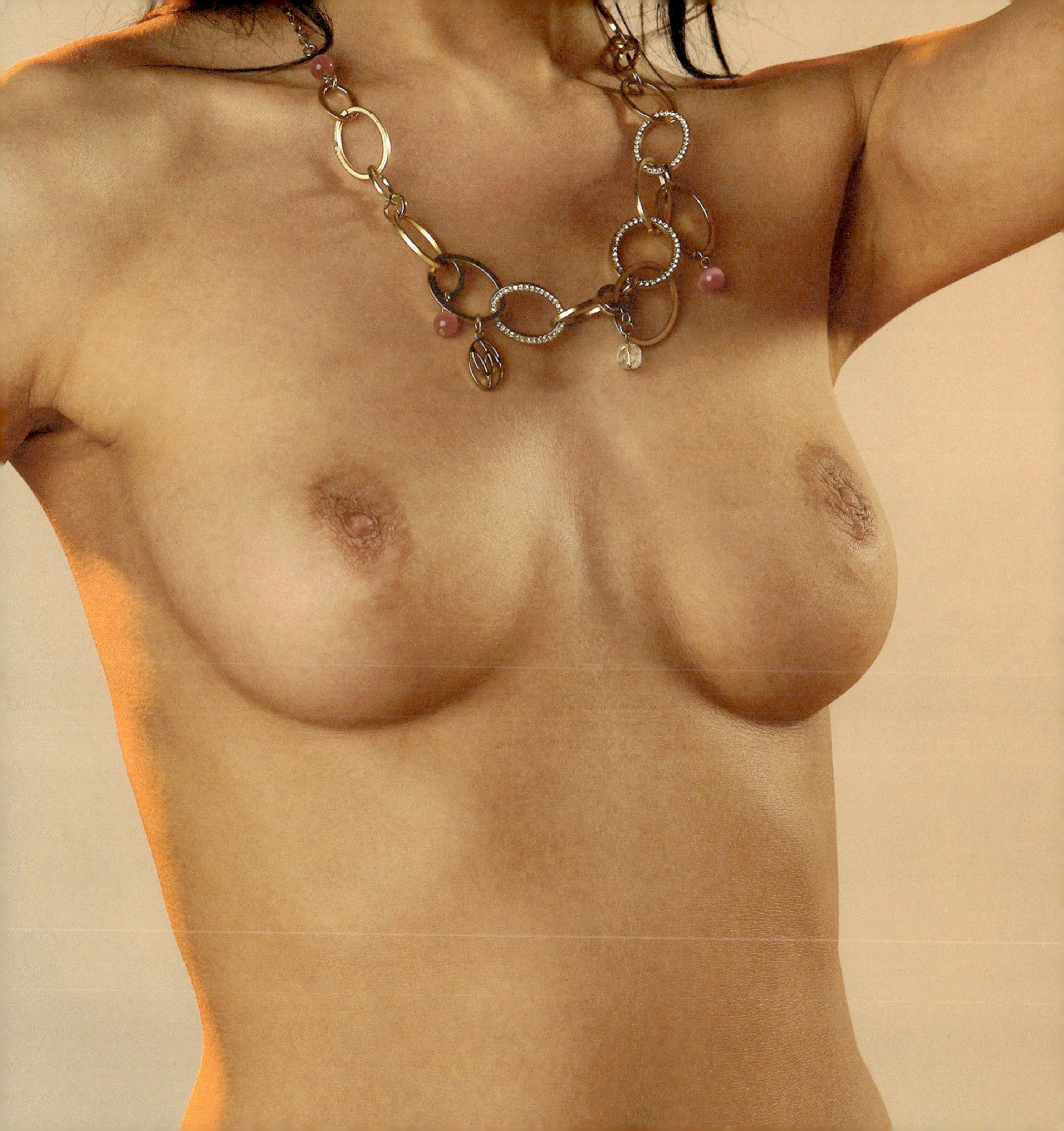

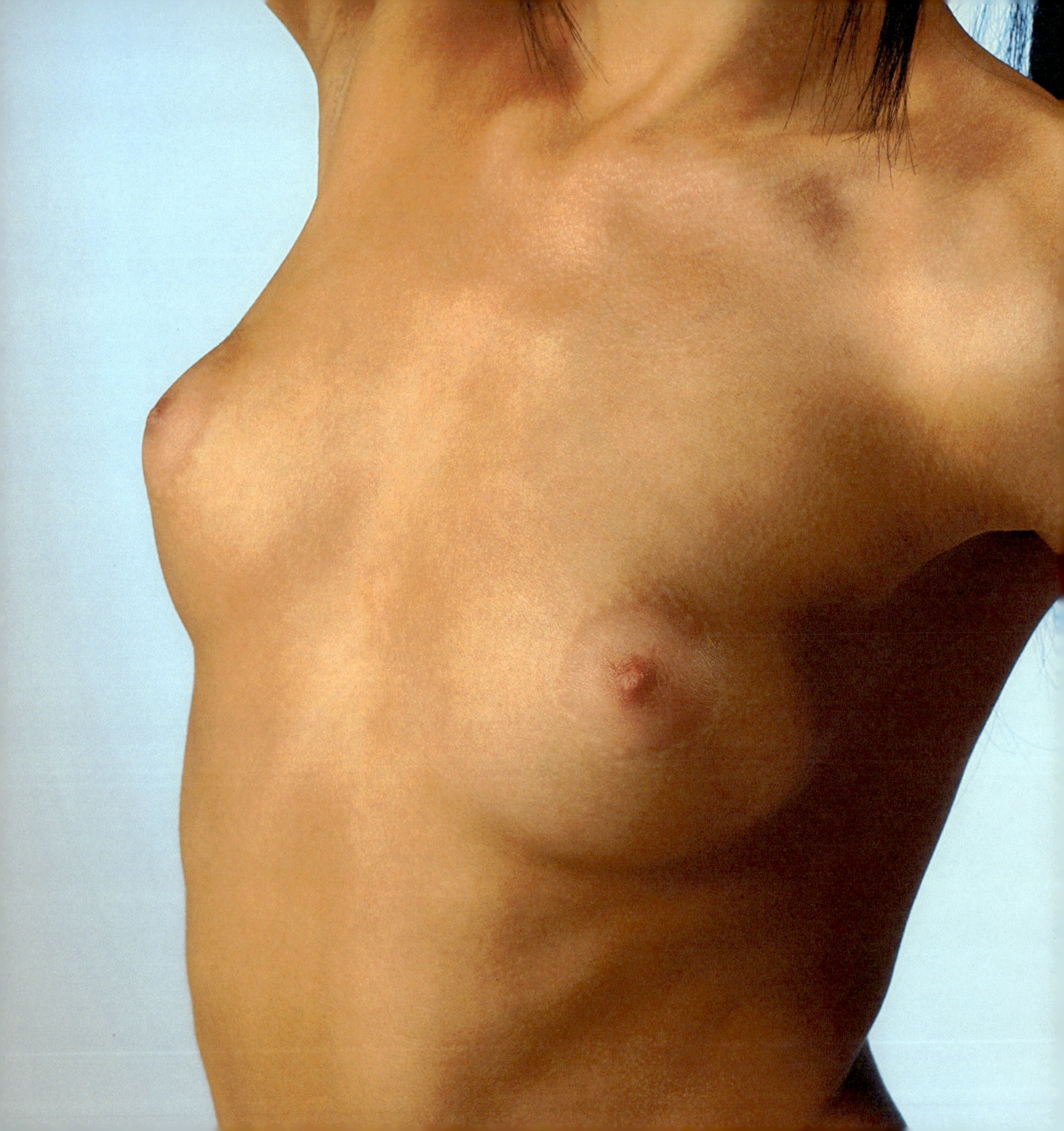

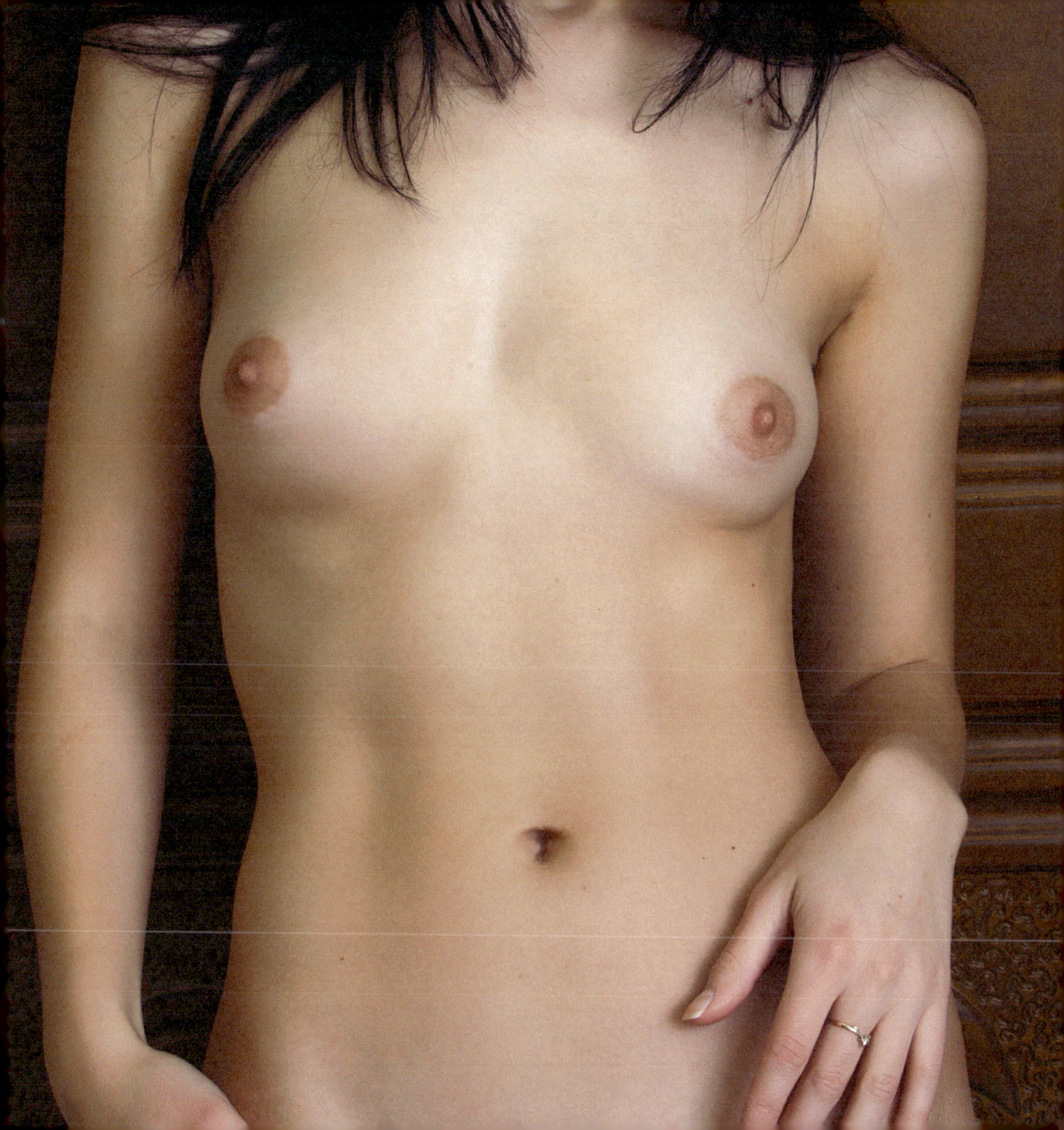

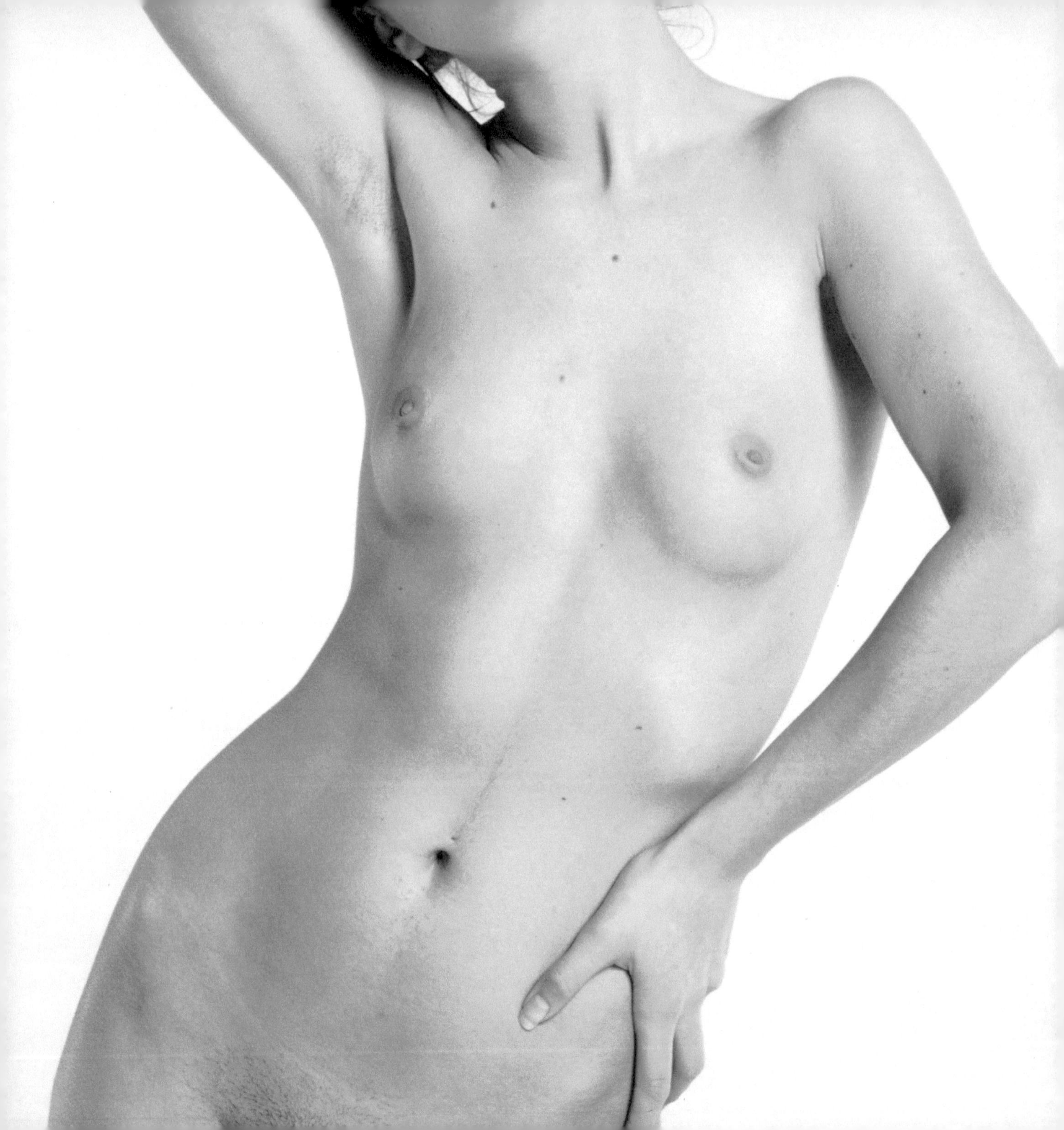

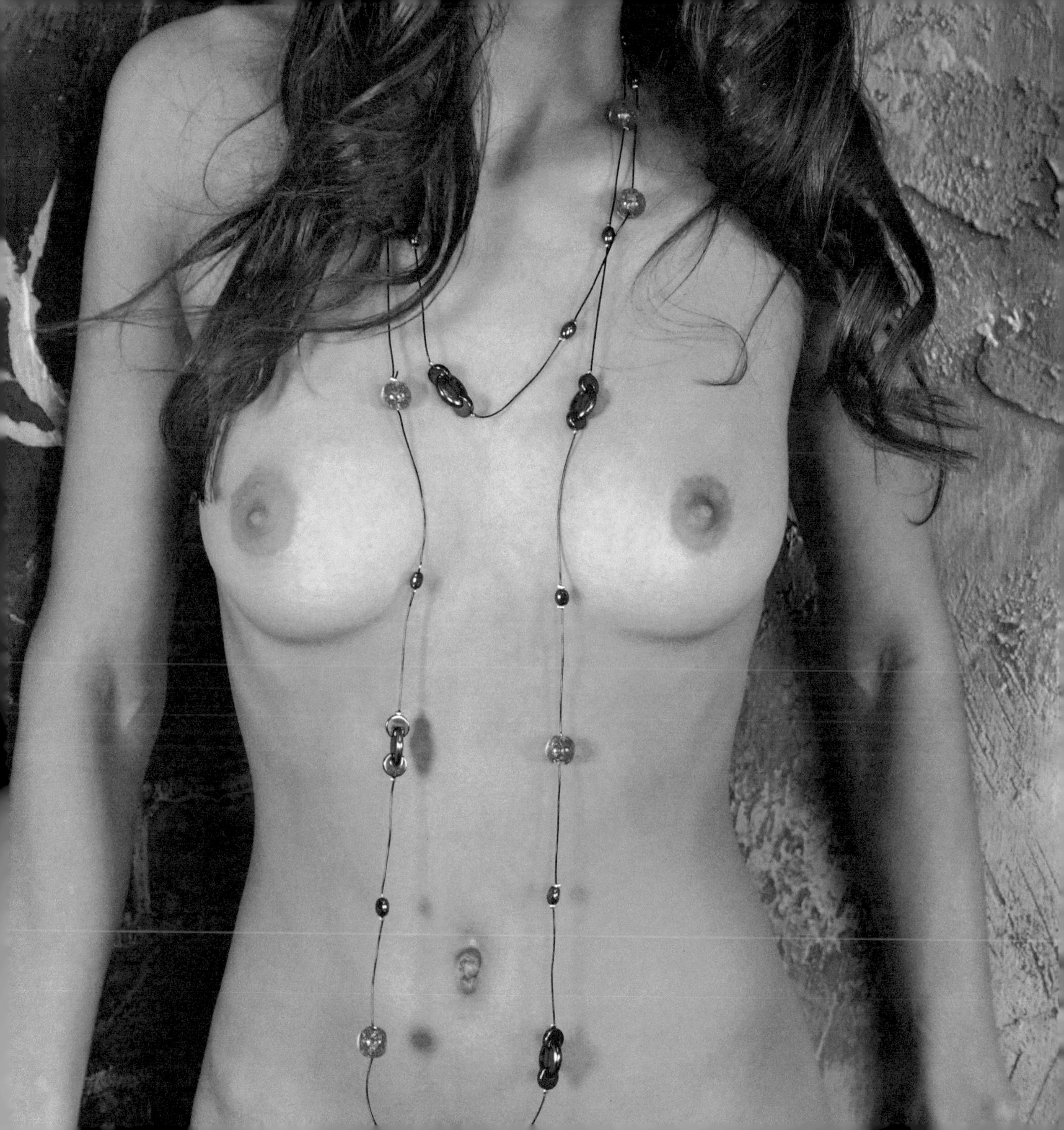

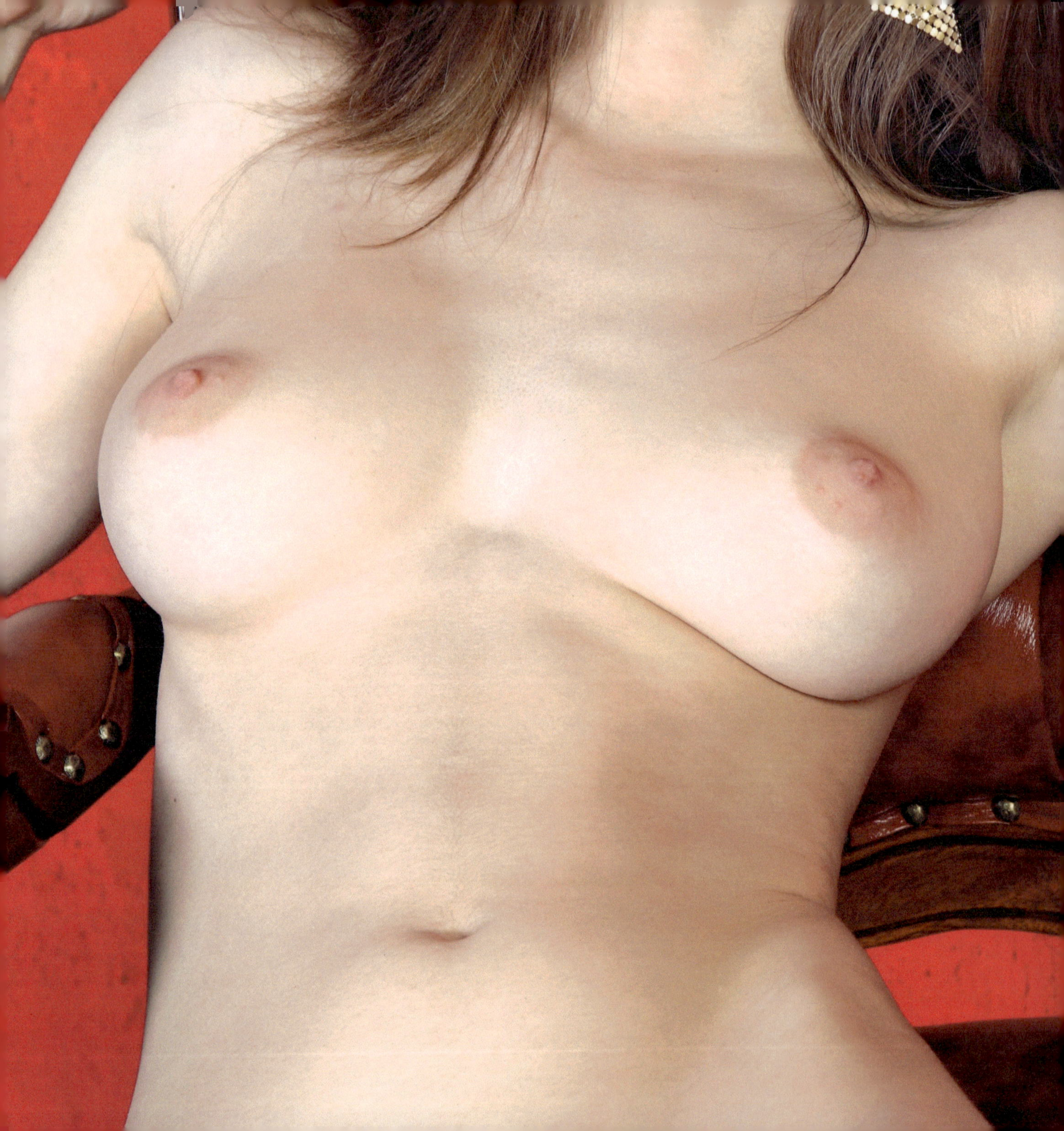

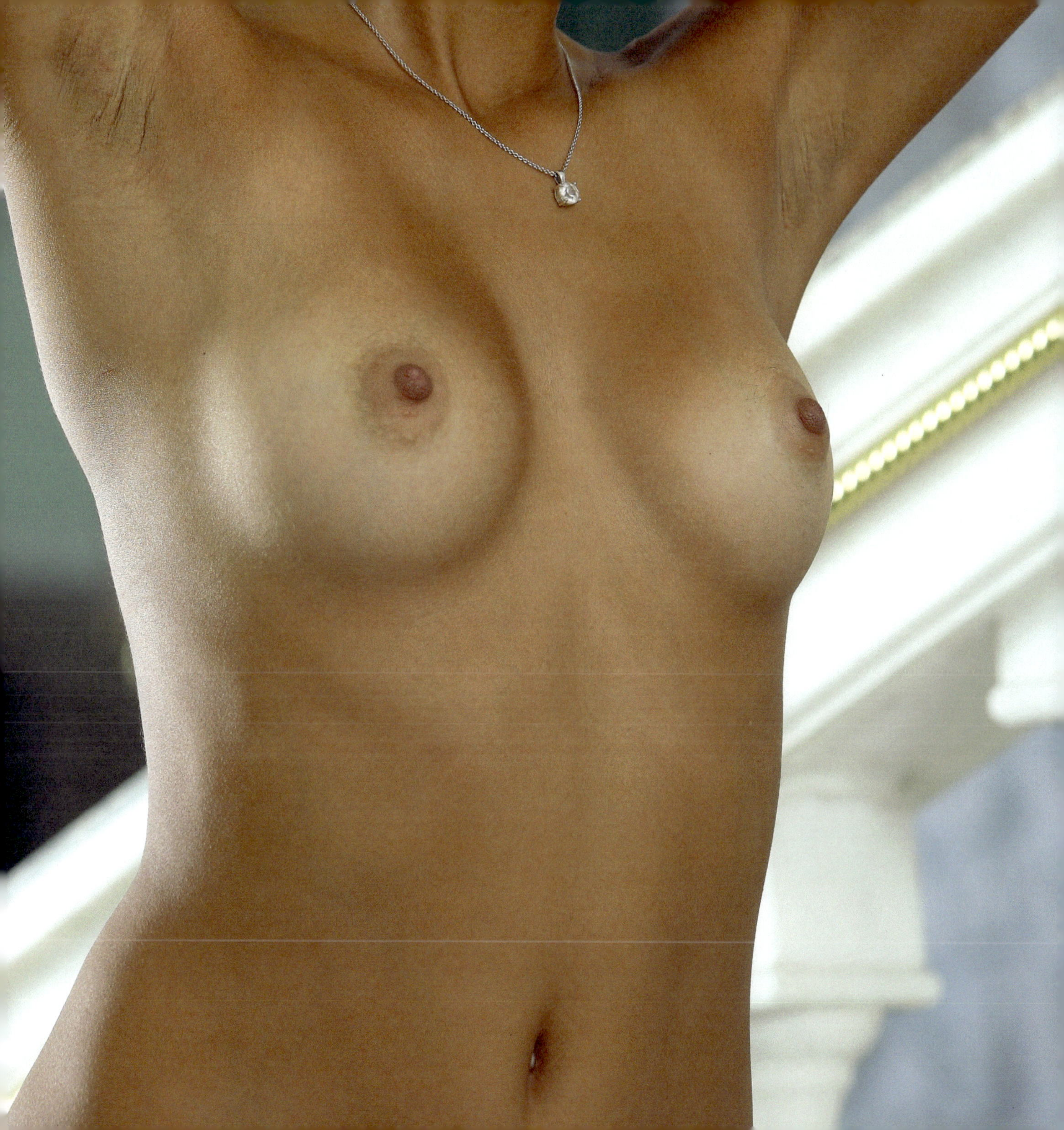

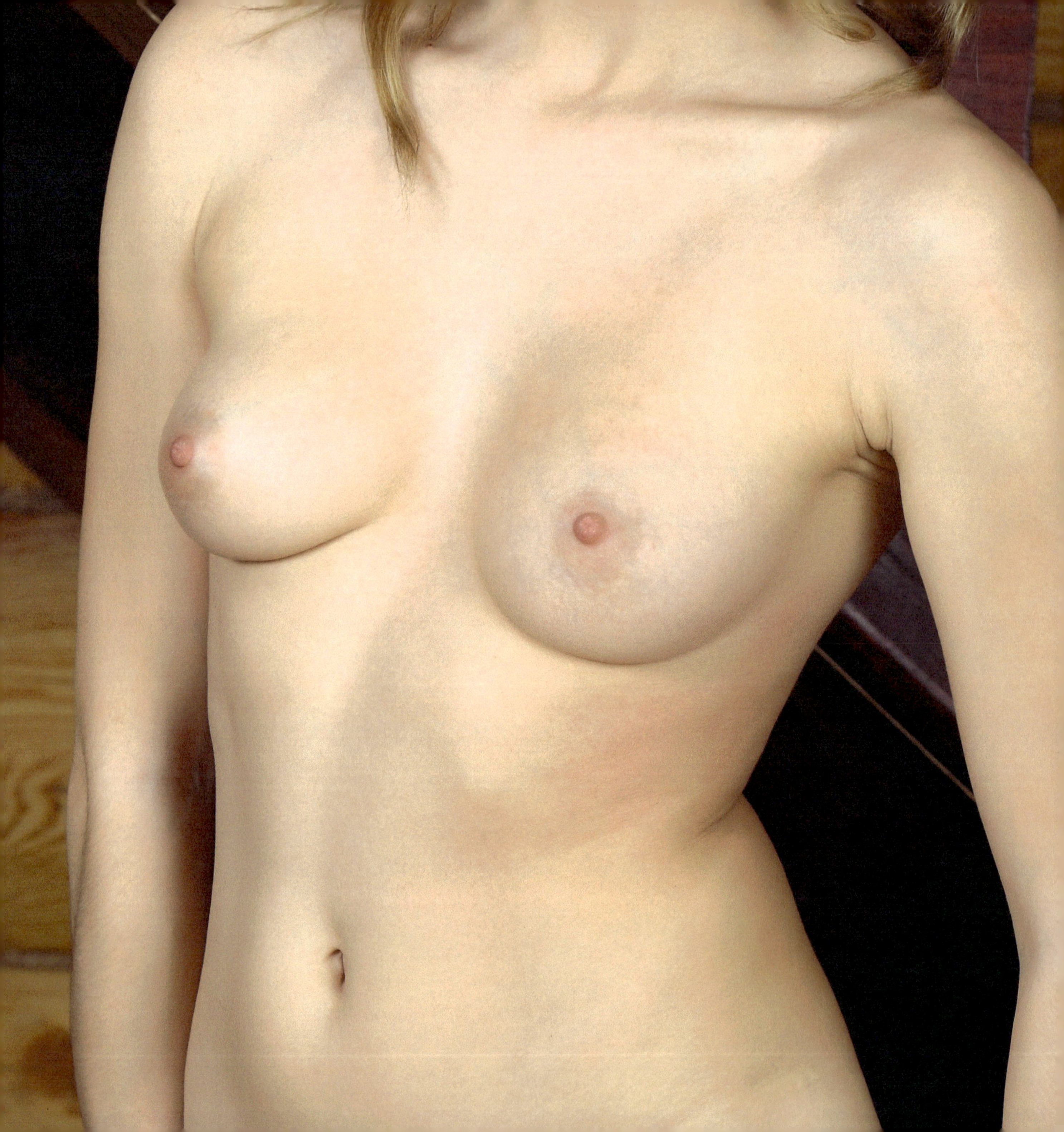

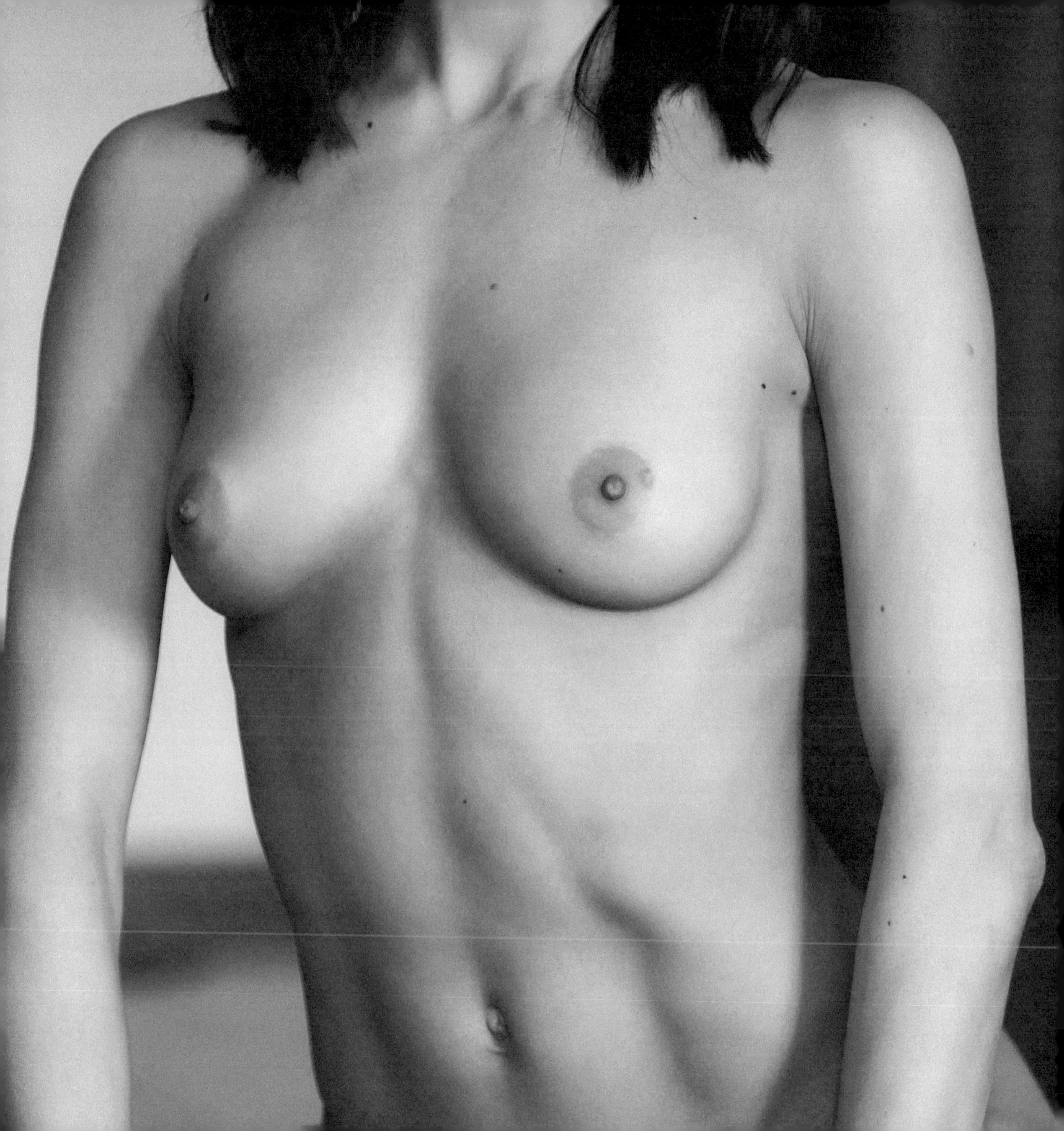

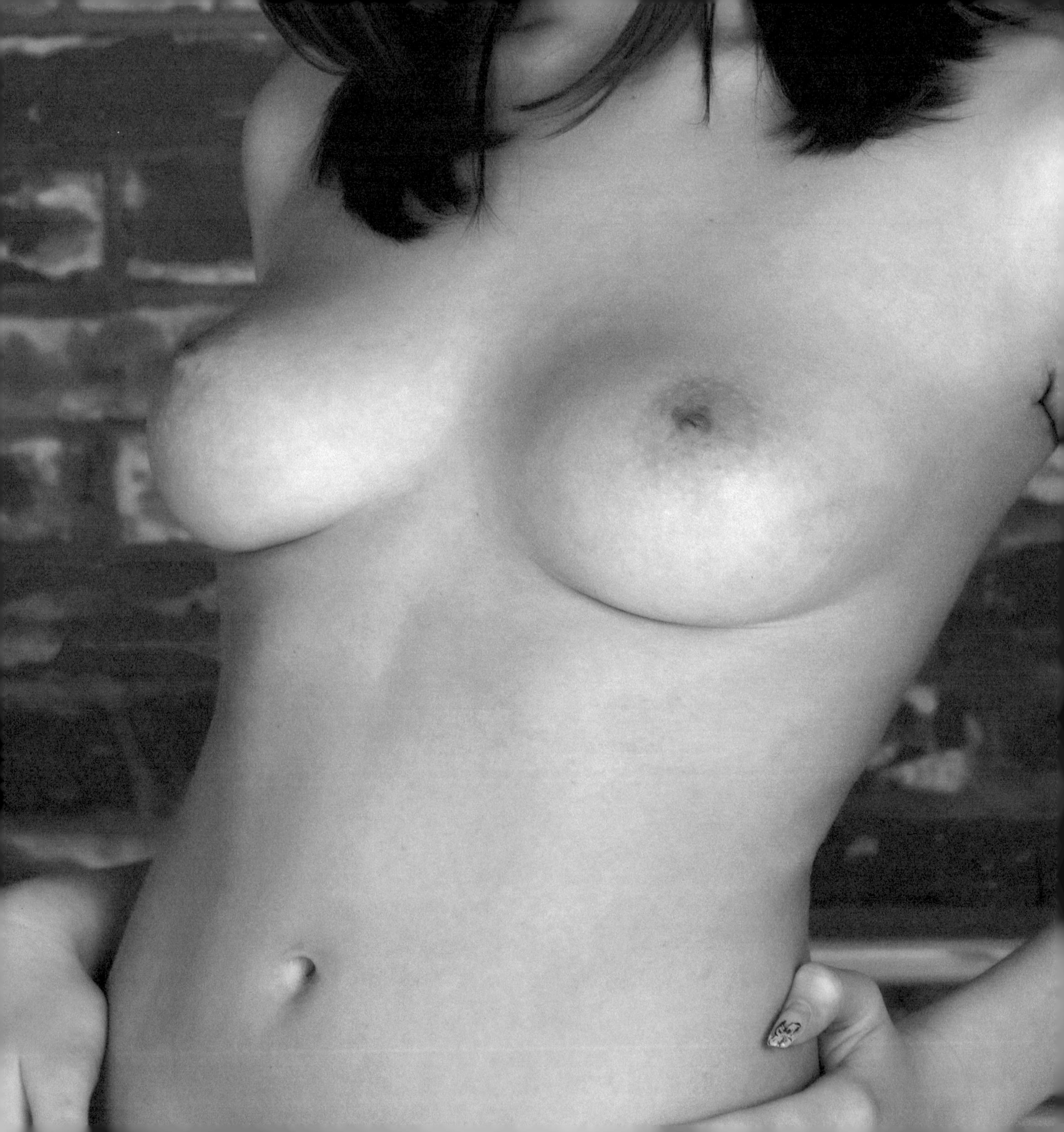

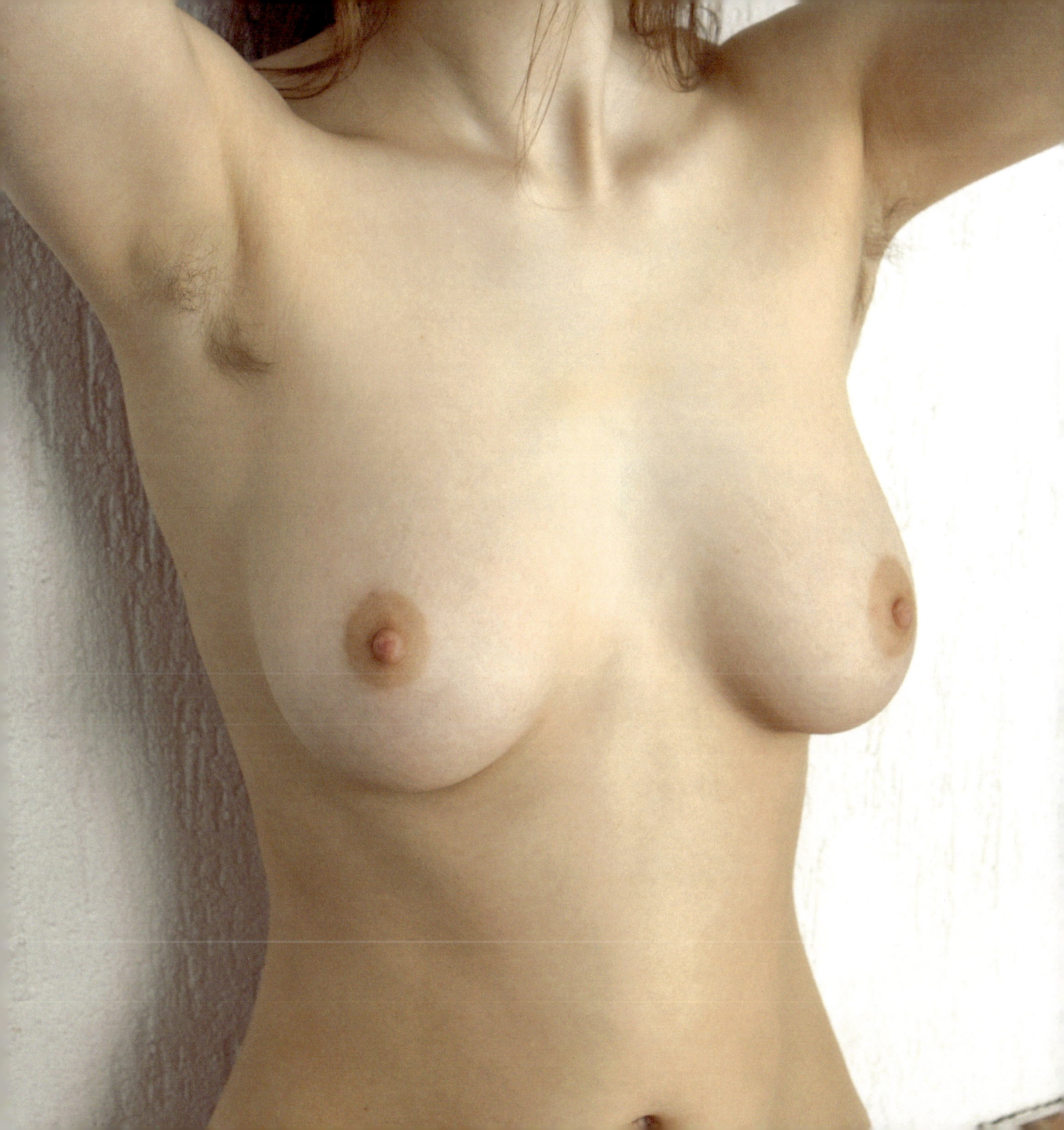

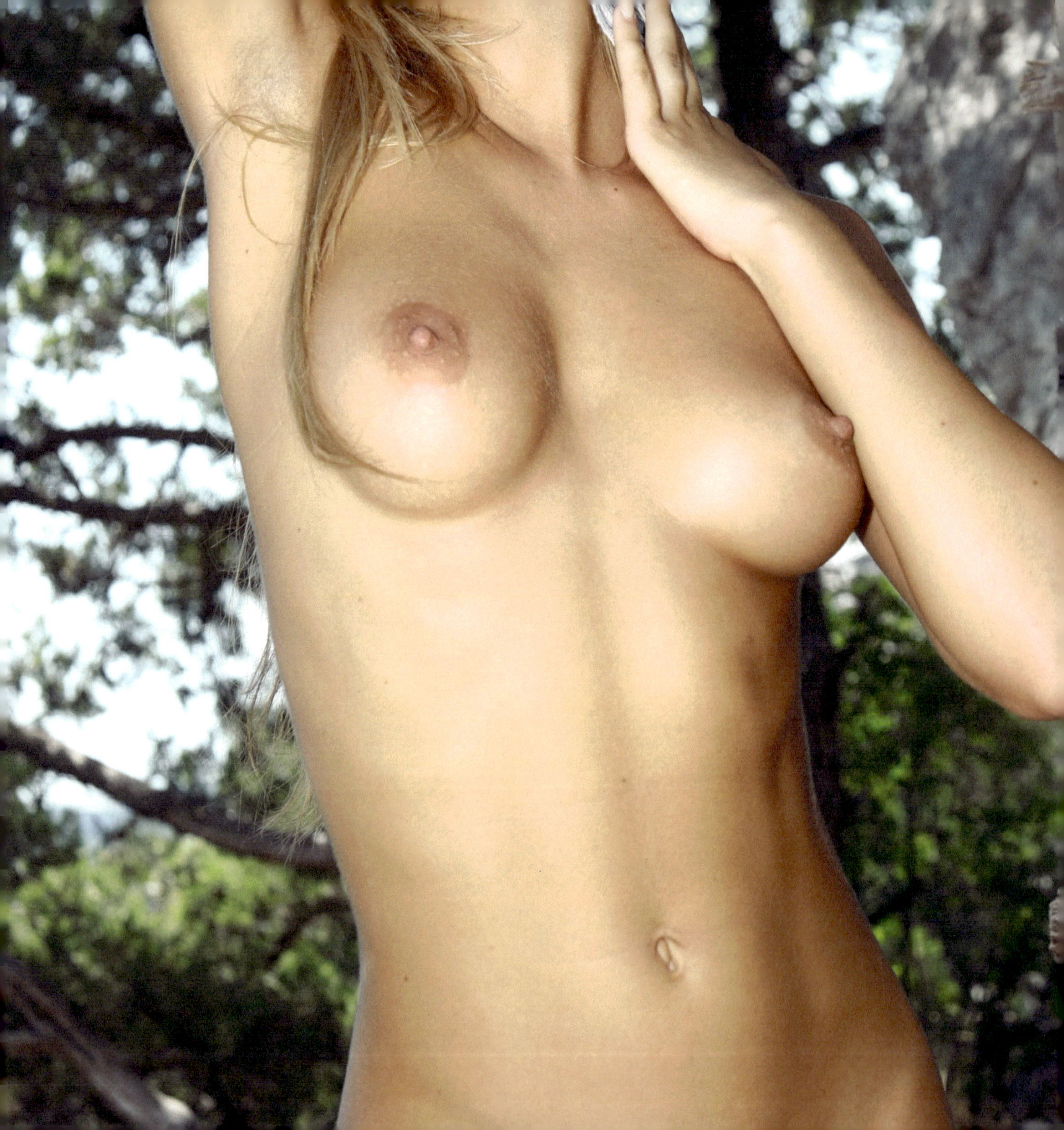

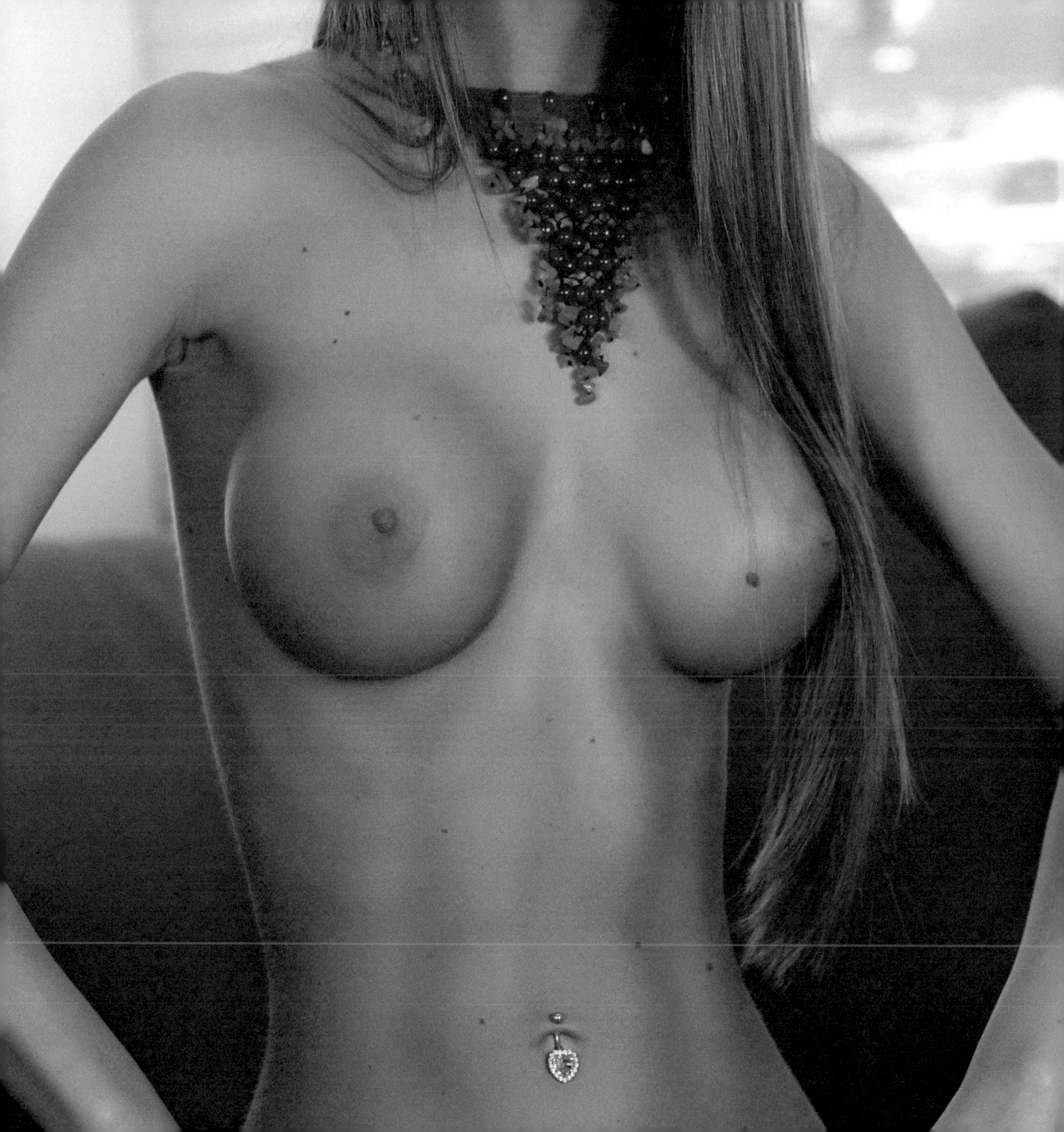

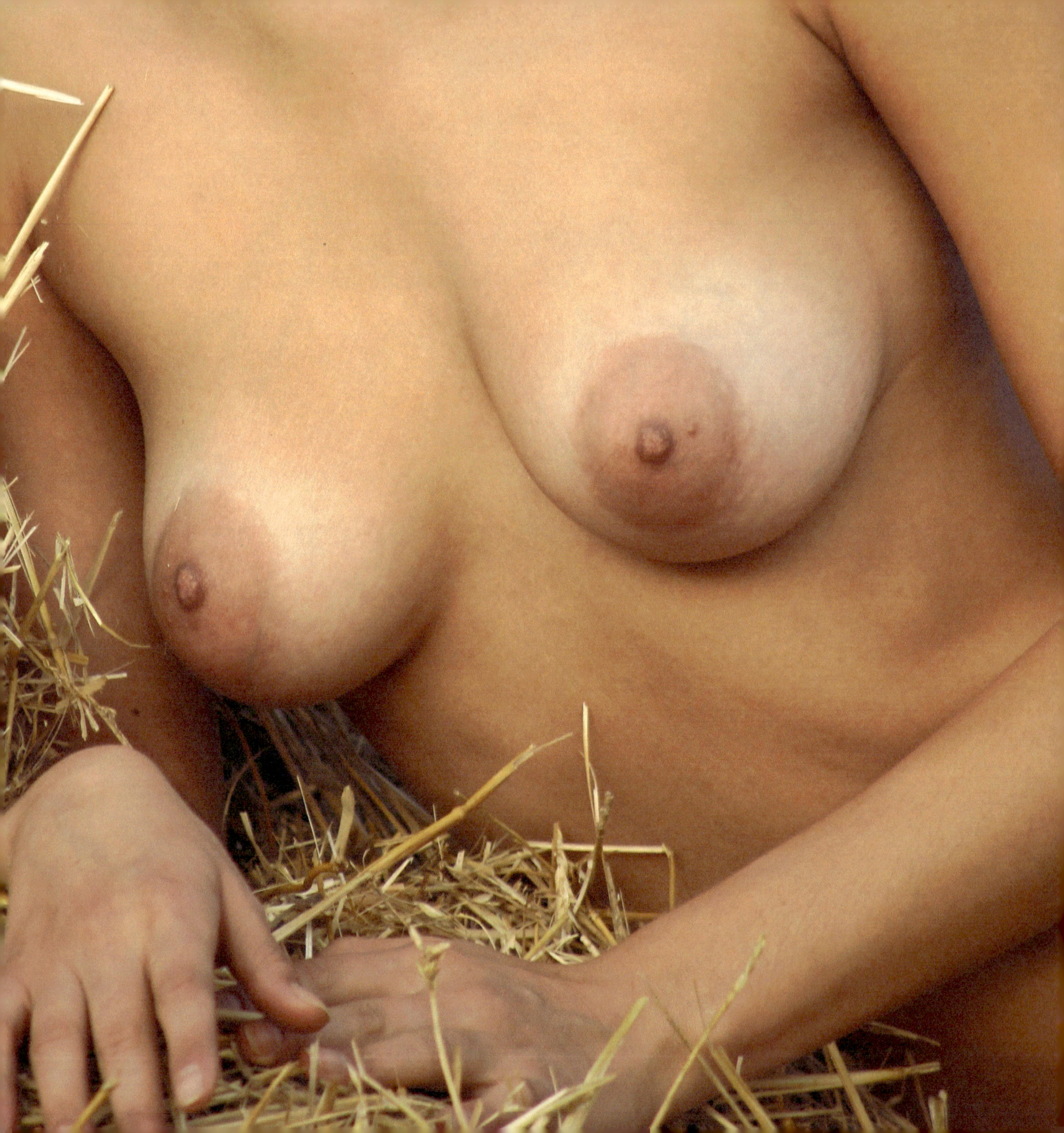

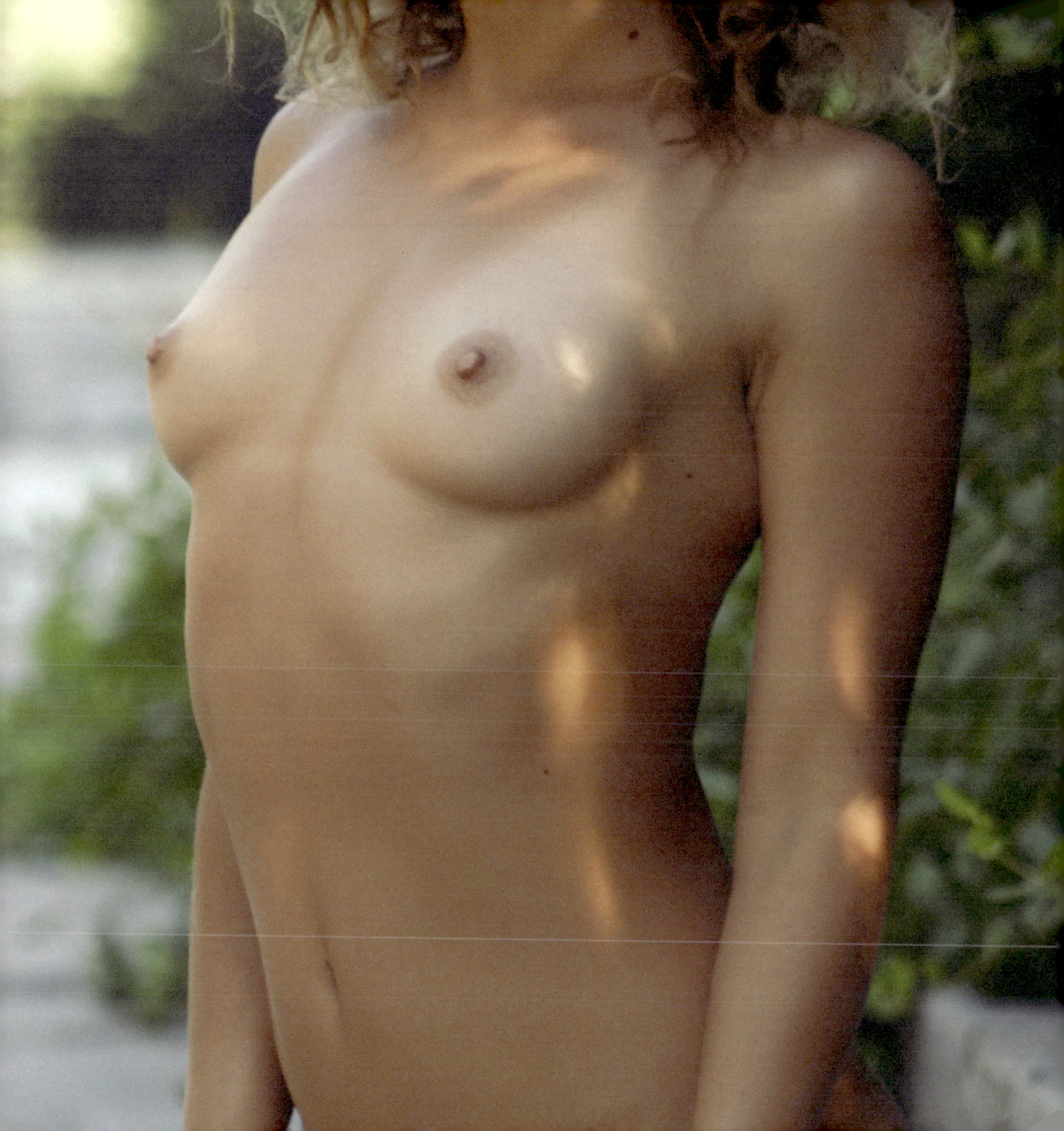

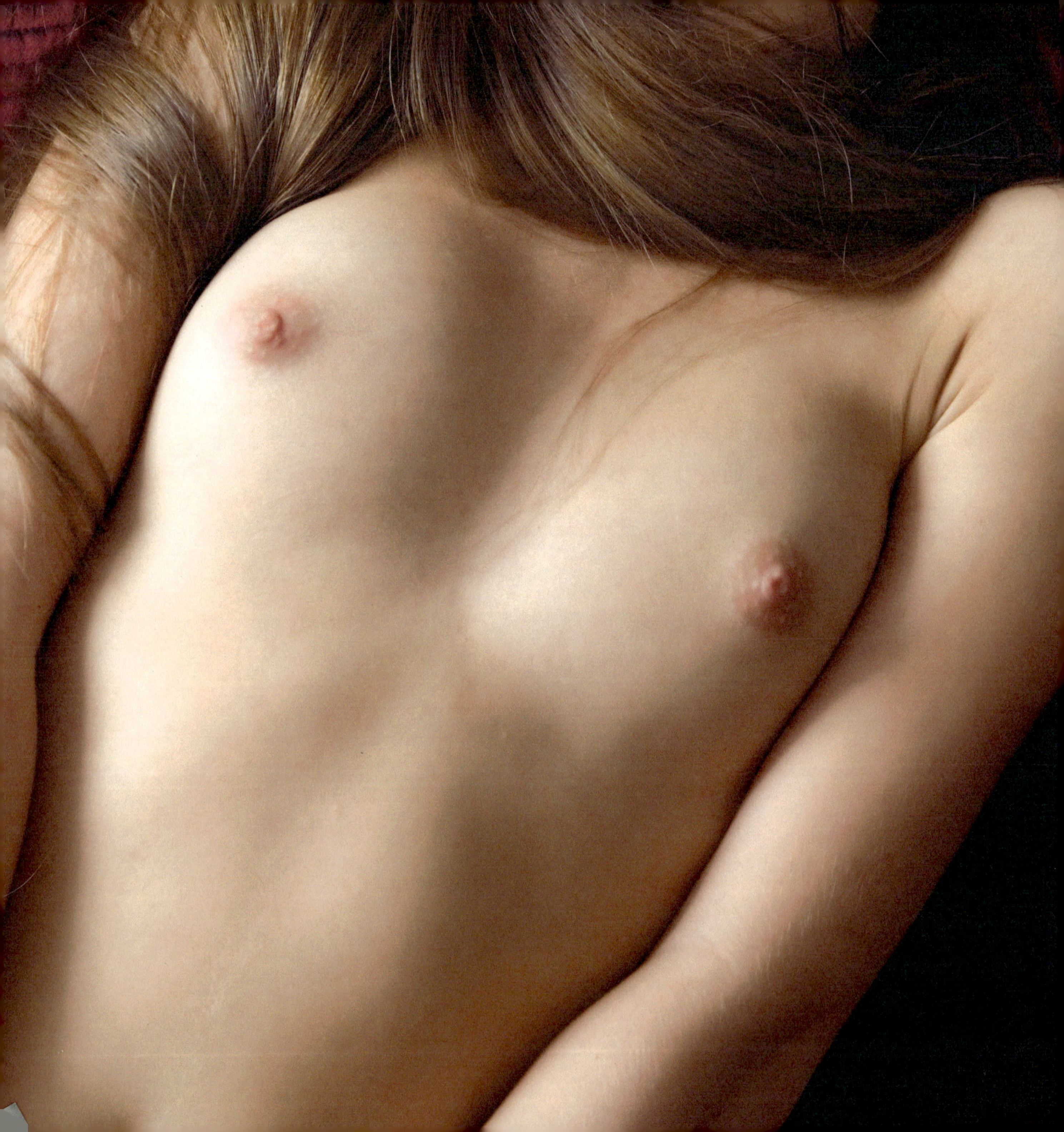

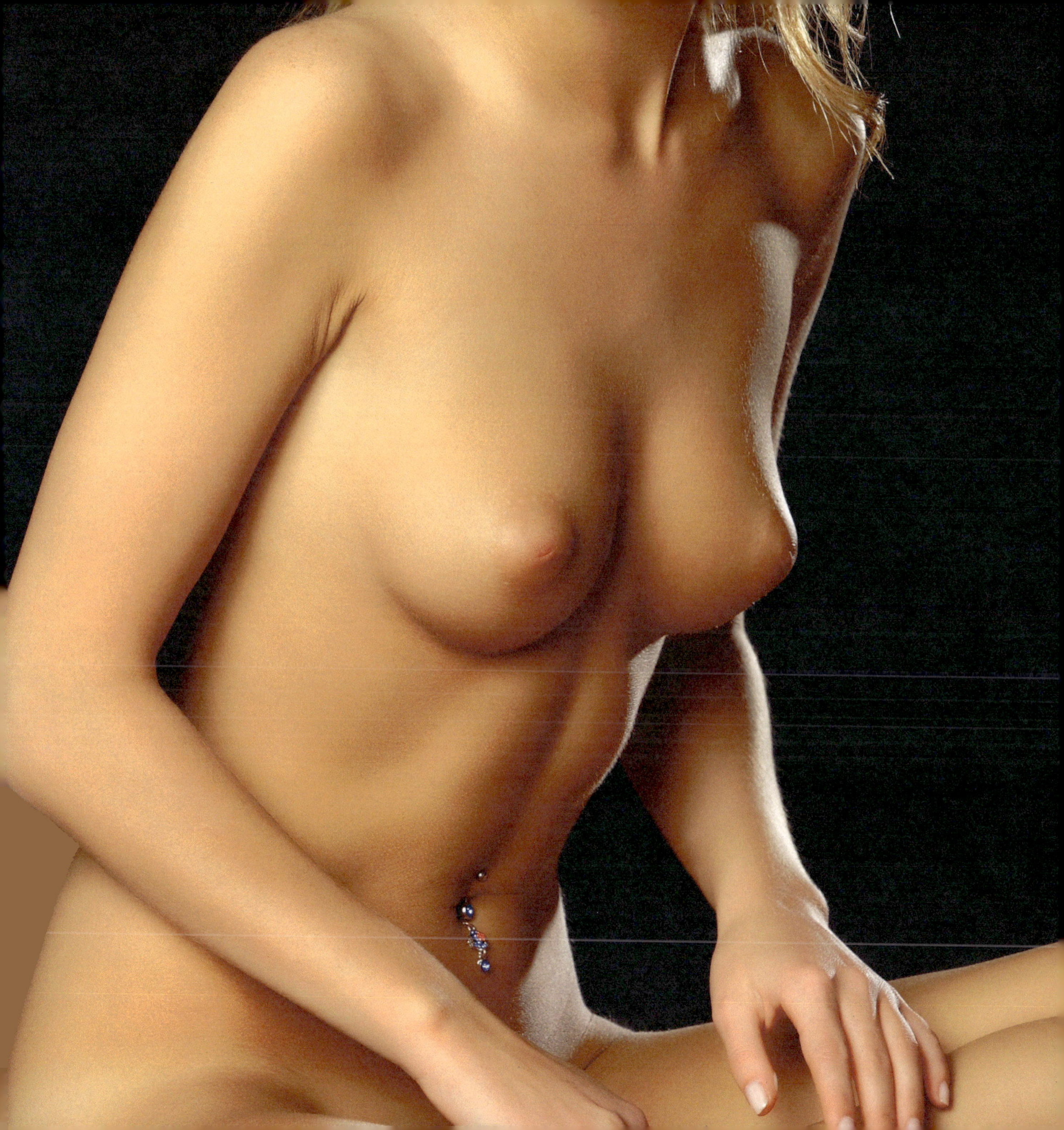

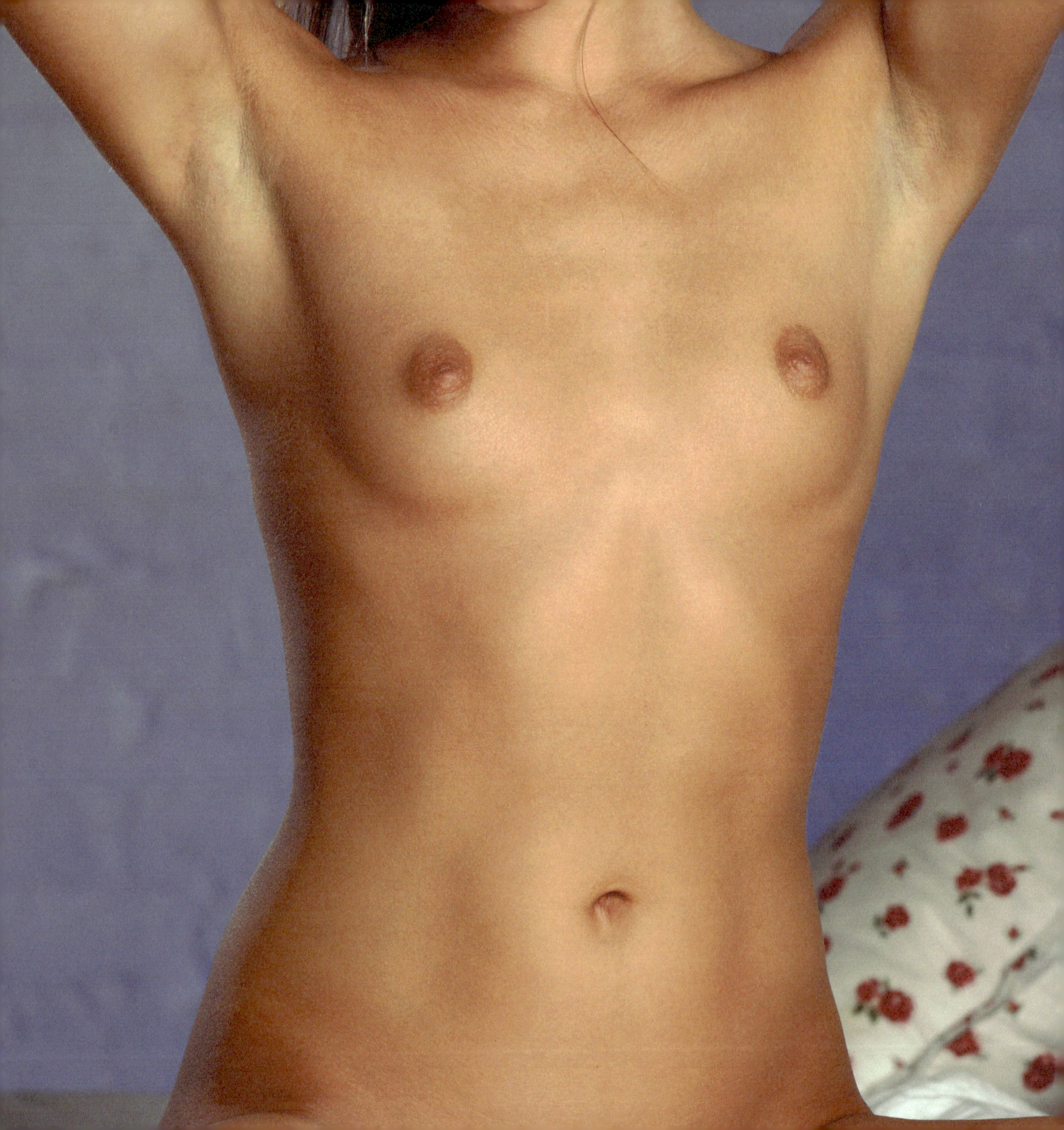

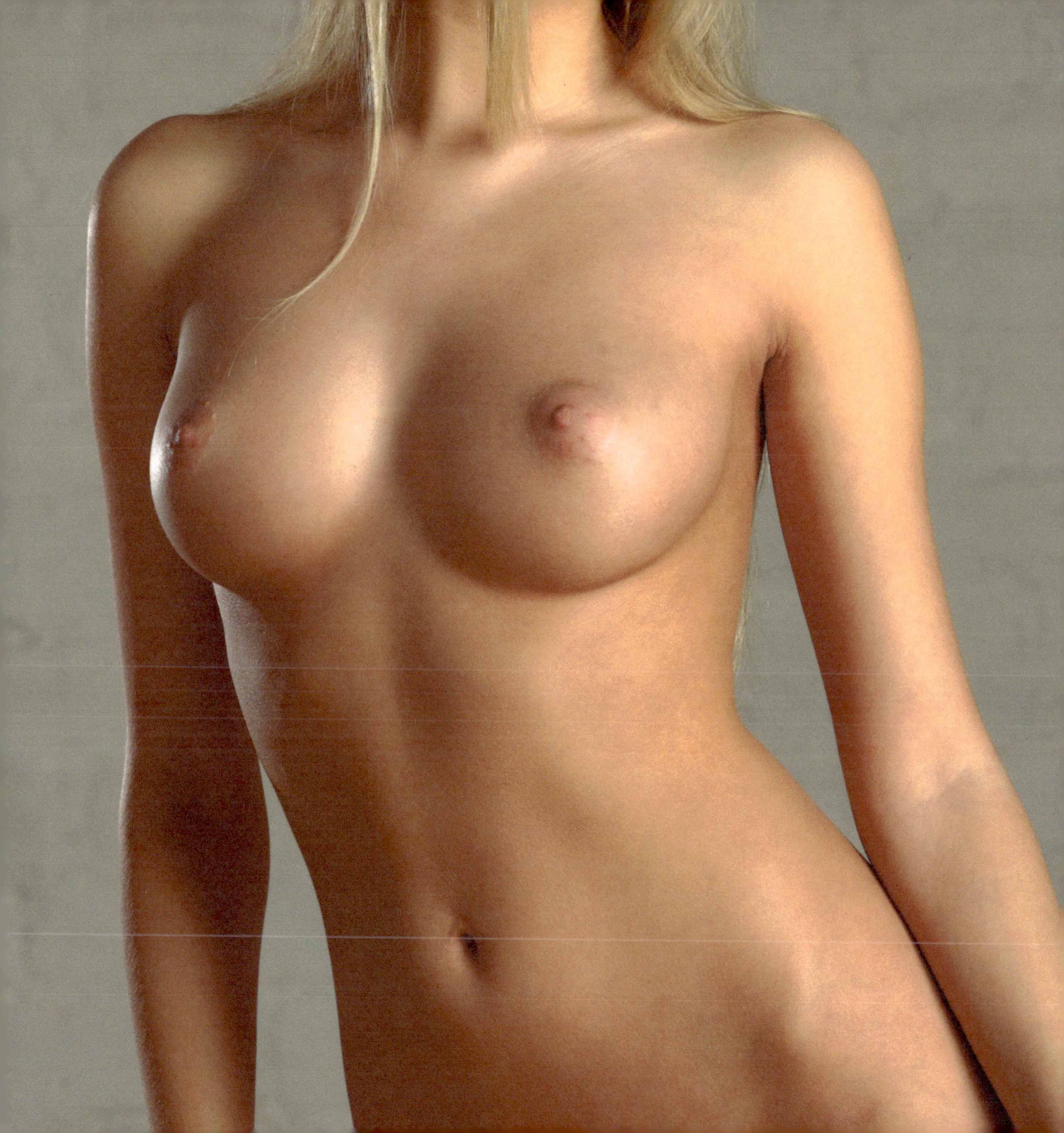

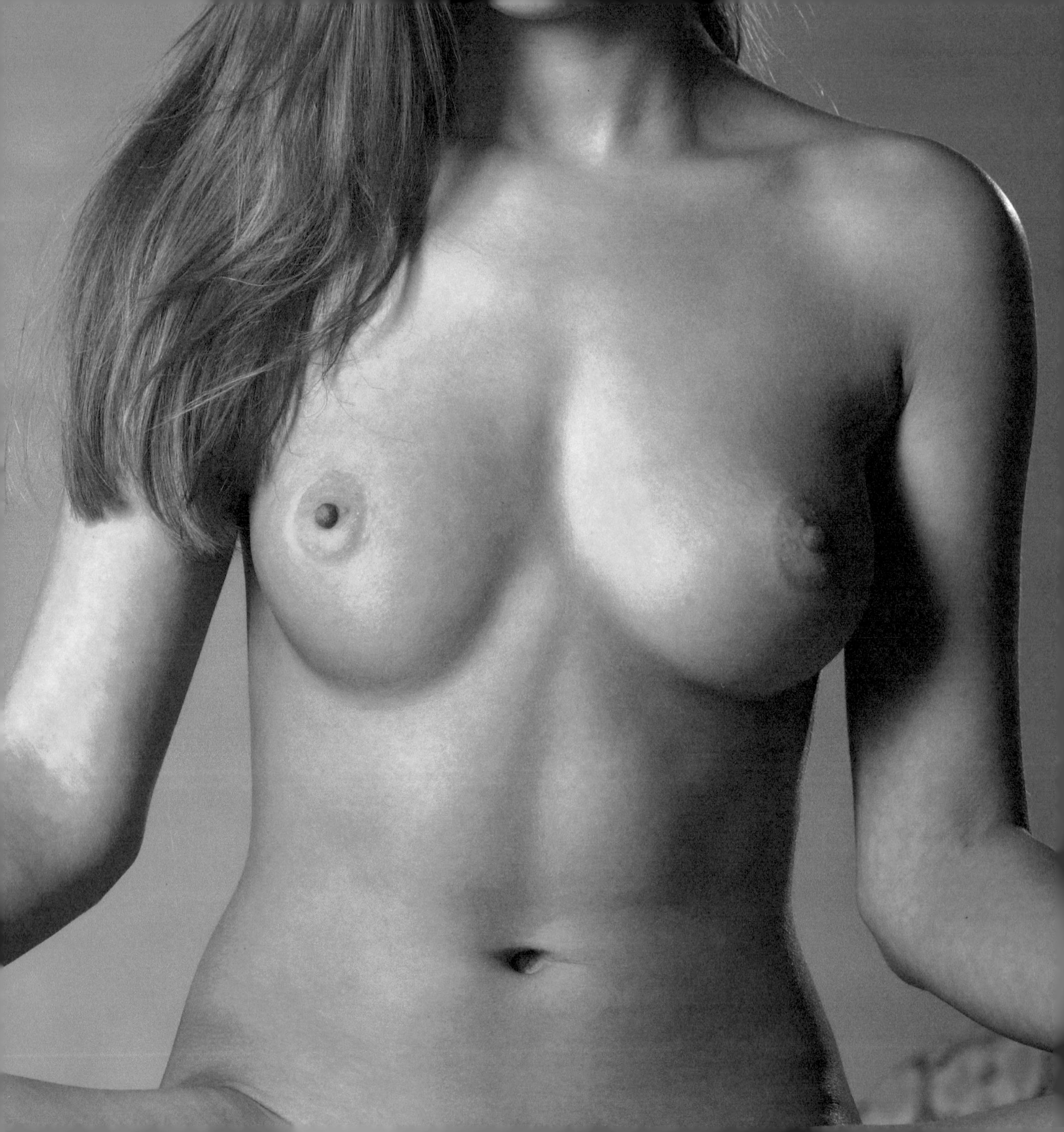

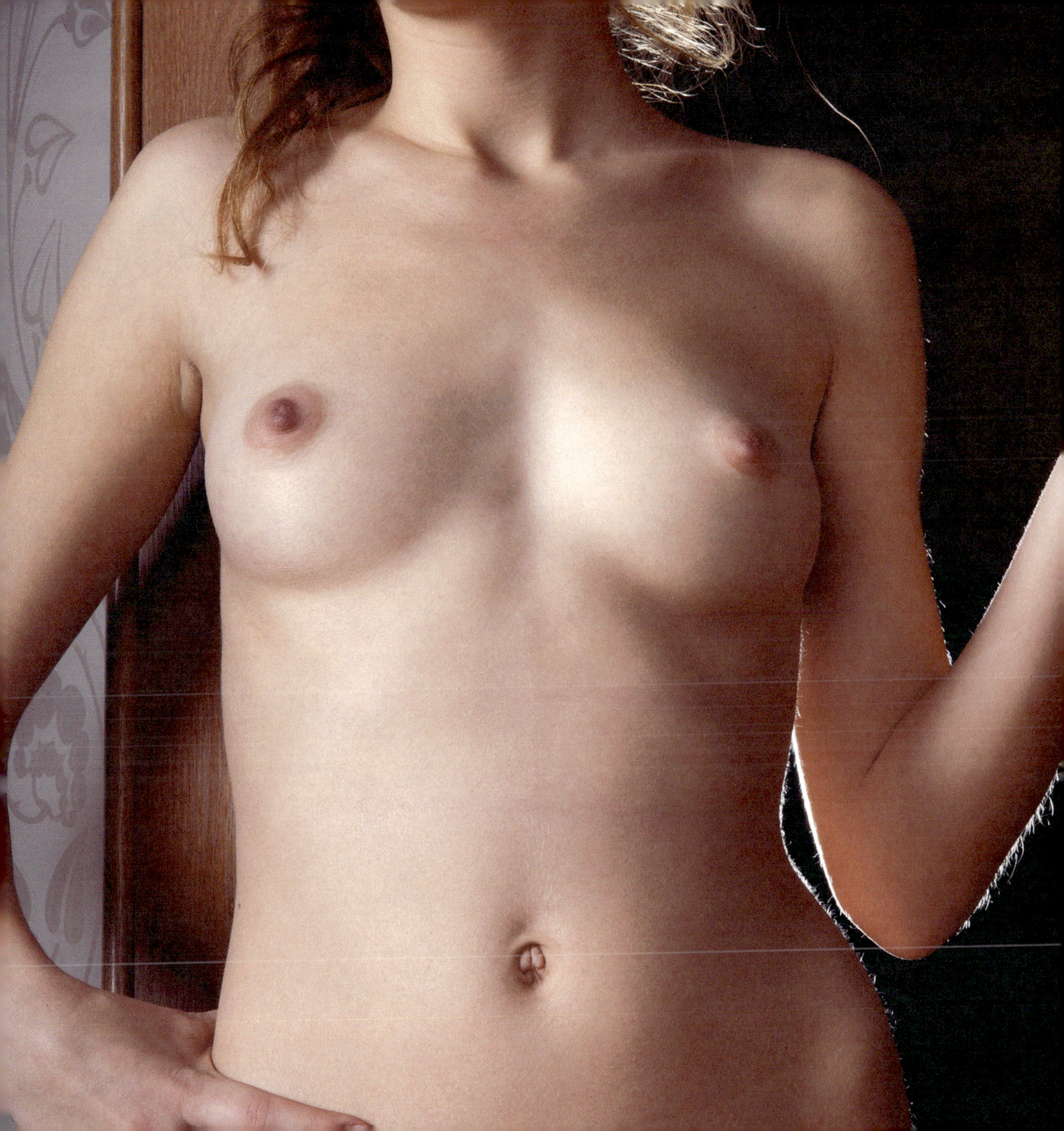

Made in the USA
Monee, IL
05 November 2026

67378005R00062